Aerobics

The Way To Fitness

Karen S. Mazzeo, M.Ed

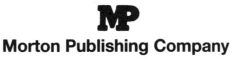

Morton Publishing Company

925 West Kenyon Avenue, Unit 12
Englewood, Colorado 80110

Typography by Ash Street Typecrafters, Inc., Denver, Colorado

Cover Design by Bob Schram, Bookends, Inc., Boulder, Colorado

Illustrations by Susan Strawn

Cover Photo and Interior Photography by Jeffrey Hall Photography, Haskins, Ohio

Copyright © 1992 by Morton Publishing Company

ISBN: 0-89582-221-0

10 9 8 7 6 5 4 3 2 1

Printed in the United States of America

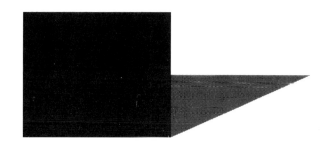

Table of Contents

CHARTS

Acknowledgments

Special appreciation is given to the following individuals who have shared their time and superb talents in this endeavor:

Robert E. Baird
Stephen I. Block
Richard W. Bowers, Ph.D.
Mary Karen Dunlap
Todd Flichel
Mary S. Garzino
Philip H. Goldstein
Jeffrey Hall
Virnette D. House
Carin Peirce Johnson
Timothy Kime II
Marian Larkin
Lauren Mangili
Katherine Marwede
Mary Beth Mazzeo
Christopher L. Mead
Douglas N. Morton
Terry L. Newman
Harold Oberhaus
Peggy Paul, R.D., L.D.
Bernard Rabin, Ed.D.
Dianne Raynor
Randy and Pam Ransom
Sue Schoonover
Kathleen Shields
Terry-Ann Spitzer
Laura Ware Babbitt

Appreciation is given to the following for granting permission to use copyrighted materials:

▶ Kenneth Cooper, M.D., M.P.H., and M. Evans Publisher, and Bantam/Doubleday/Dell

▶ R.V. Hockey and Times/Mirror Mosby College Publishing

▶ Werner W.K. Hoeger, Ph.D., and Morton Publishing Company

▶ The National Dairy Council and The Oregon Dairy Council

A special thank you to the following companies for providing apparel and equipment with which to photograph:

▶ Nike, Incorporated, One Bowerman Drive, Beaverton, OR 97005 (1-800-535-6453) for women's fitness apparel.

▶ Kevin Schaack, Manager, Foot Locker - Bowling Green Mall (Ohio) (419-354-0567) for Nike Aerobic and Cross-Trainer Shoes.

▶ Sports Step, Inc., for The Step and instructional videos. For additional information on The Step, please call Sports Step, Inc. (1-800-SAY-STEP).

▶ SPRI Products, Inc., 507 N. Wolf Road, Wheeling, IL 60090 (1-800-222-7774) for rubber resistance bands and tubing.

Dedication

To all of the people who serve as role models of personal excellence to others, continually expressing the unique talents they've been given, and who've personally been an inspiration to me to pursue my own natural talents

- ▶ Dick — my best friend and husband for twenty-six years, whose consistent values and commitment to maintaining high standards is a daily joy to experience.
- ▶ Mary Beth — for her relentless dedication to all the dimensions of physical fitness and mental training.
- ▶ Michael — whose natural creativity in problem-solving is absolutely second to none!
- ▶ Phil, Lauren and Virnette — who serve as tremendous role models in both their professional careers and fitness endeavors.
- ▶ John — for his continual sharing of invitational methods of teaching and presenting wellness ideas — a true "master teacher."
- ▶ Terry — whose personal support of my talents is totally appreciated and whose ability to inspire others toward the fitness lifestyle is a joy to behold.
- ▶ Ed — for his powerful communication skills which have greatly enriched my Christian spiritual life.
- ▶ "JimRob" — who has naturally instilled the winning mindset in his athletes all the years I've known him.
- ▶ Anne — my favorite author, whose philosophies about living have inspired my teaching, my writing, and my daily life.
- ▶ Doug — who knows how to motivate and encourage his authors at key times, in very supporting ways.
- ▶ Peter — whose openness to tapping into his unlimited potential has given me the needed inspiration to continue to pursue the answers to "the winning-mindset mosiac."

Thanks to each of you for serving as my needed role-models of personal excellence, enabling me to pursue my own unlimited potential!

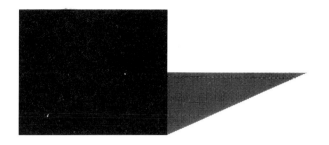

Introduction

The fitness activities entitled Aerobics (also called exercise-dance) and Step Training (which uses a 4–12" step bench), together, are currently two of the hottest, most popular methods used today for achieving and maintaining physical fitness. Aerobics has enjoyed two decades of unbelievable success and Step Training, although a relatively new activity, is rapidly attaining the same highly acclaimed distinction as *the* way to fitness!

With two such unique and powerful success stories, it is understandable that a quality, informative, course-oriented text describing the basic principles, techniques, and vast possible combinations of each is needed. *Aerobics•The Way To Fitness* has been developed for fitness enthusiasts to fill that dual-need. Since the text is designed primarily for the novice, complete explanations for developing a personalized program are given, in an easy to follow, sequential learning order.

An invitation to develop the mindset for a fitness lifestyle sets the stage for this exciting new comprehensive First Edition text. Understanding the mindset process and what makes up the self-management model, and how to use each for change, is described in Chapter 1.

Chapter 2 puts definition to the vast terminologies we use such as one's total fitness, physical fitness, aerobics, aerobic exercise, aerobic dance, intensity, safe training zone (or target heart rates), impact (low/power low/high/combo), plyometrics, and the training effect. It provides the foundation from which to build the physical fitness techniques you choose to use.

Chapter 3 gets your program underway by establishing where you are, today! Testing procedures for

all of the key components of physical fitness are given, and charts are provided for you to describe your starting points. You can, therefore, set goals that you choose, and will have the ability to monitor your progress and see your results as they occur.

Chapter 4 presents the basic building blocks — the principles — for developing your own aerobics and step training programs. The four program segments, which include the warm up/aerobic activity/strength training/ and cool down-flexibility training-relaxation phase/, are each described. Principles for using the popular elastic bands and tubing are also given. To add variety to your aerobics (or step training) and strength training phases, ideas on how to perform interval aerobics combining both, is presented.

To answer the many questions asked by individuals with special needs and concerns, Chapter 5 is included. It lists possible program challenges or problem areas, and then solutions to consider.

Chapter 6 places an emphasis on the initial consideration of any physical fitness experience — safety — which is encouraged with proper body positioning (i.e., posture). Since good positioning, especially of the spine and joints, underlies all physical movement that you'll ever choose to do, this chapter is paramount, and where the techniques of your physical fitness program must begin.

Chapter 7 presents many techniques you can use in your program segments from start to finish, through numerous photographs. Included are:

▶ Basic aerobics steps and gestures for each of the four program phases;

▶ The five basic bench approaches, correct step training postures, and basic step training patterns, including several popular variations;

▶ Techniques for using the rubber elastic bands and tubing, and hand-held weights, both alone or in conjunction with the bench.

You will notice that the exercise movements have all been described and then photographed using a "mirrored" method. The student will easily understand that a movement described and visualized as using the *left* foot/arm/or side of the body is actually the *right* foot/arm/side of the model (see Figure I.1). Thus the student does not have to reverse the direction of what is pictured and what is performed! You simply perform the movement on the same side of the body as you see it photographed and described.

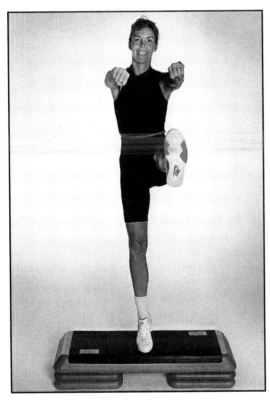

Figure I.1. Stepping up onto the bench, taking weight on your *left* foot, kick your *right* leg forward, waist-high.

Chapter 8 takes apart the *how to* of both aerobics and step training choreography, for the pre-planning on your part that must be considered, in order for you to independently develop your own personalized program, or when directing others. You'll find the possibilities for using a variety of movement are unlimited.

Chapter 9, presents the principles of stress management and follows with relaxation techniques. Understanding creative ways to rejuvenate your mental and physical energy immediately following exercise is the revitalizing touch needed for the final segment of the physical fitness workout. The techniques can be used for other portions of your day, too, when relaxation is the missing link needed to regain *balance.*

Complimenting all of the information on exercise and energy expenditure, is Chapter 10, which focuses on the intake of energy — your diet, current nutritional concerns, and weight management strategies. It concludes with a ranking of fitness priorities and the establishment of total program goals.

The text includes an Appendix of charts, which can be used for monitoring change or developing specific skills, and are perforated for easy removal for class or instructor evaluation. For your convenience, an Index of key topics is also included. Enjoy the process of developing the mindset and actions for a lifetime of fitness.

You are the master of your ship.
Nothing, and no one else,
can do it for you.

NOTE TO INSTRUCTORS:
When you teach as shown and described in this text, realize that when you cue "weight on *left* foot," you, the instructor, are (as the model is) actually on your own *right* foot.

Chapter 1

Developing A Mindset For The Fitness Lifestyle

The value of time
The virtue of patience
The success of perseverance
The influence of example
The improvement of talent
The joy of creativity!
. . . I reflect upon each of these,
while I work out.
Slowly, I begin to realize that
there is nothing more challenging,
than working to develop the fitness
of my mind and flesh.
When I am successful, it establishes
a permanent MINDSET,
"a confidence"
that allows me to do well
in everything else I try!

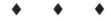

"I'm gonna live forever!" is a key line from a popular song of a few years ago. These words represent a programmed belief, or mindset, that most of us can readily identify with today, primarily because we thoroughly believe it about ourselves. Consequently, the majority of us (no matter what age we are) act accordingly and live our lives as if this quote were true.

Strongly believing in our physical immortality, we seem to routinely disregard any rational self-discipline we might have when it comes to our physical well-being. If the moment dictates that we

should enjoy the good life by overeating and underexercising, many times we give in and just "go for it!" Our internal dialogue, or the external comments of others, tells us "Why not? You only live once. Enjoy!"

Have you ever wondered: Where does this current, prevailing mindset that many of us hold onto — this mindset of immortality, that we are going to live forever, at least in the physical sense — originate? It is important to ask this type of question of oneself at the beginning of a fitness course because it represents becoming more aware of the mindset process — aware of all of the unique factors fueling our choices. When we consider not only the individual behaviors we express but also *what factors lie behind these actions* — the emotional forces, the attitudes, the beliefs, and the programming already present and operating our "mental computers," we can then understand fitness for a lifetime and have it become the programmed belief (mindset) we consistently choose.

First, we must understand the steps of the fascinating process we go through — in a split second — when we are asked to make an immediate choice relative to our daily lifestyle. ("Shall we take the stairs, or ride the elevator up the two flights to the classroom/office today?") Examining the steps of the mindset process is an exciting first step for developing positive change in any poor habits we are willing to change. Healthy lifestyle choices are like time-honored recipes that contain key ingredients used in a unique order for consistent good results.

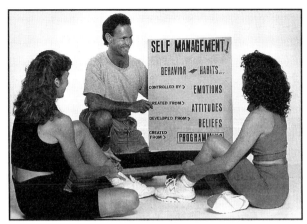

Figure 1.1. The process of developing a mindset for the fitness lifestyle includes becoming more aware of 1) the choices we constantly make, and 2) what internal resources we've used to make these choices.

AWARENESS OF YOUR CHOICES (i.e., BEHAVIOR/ACTIONS/HABITS)

Whatever we prefer to call it — behavior, actions, or habits — our choices are the end result of a unique problem-solving strategy we have within ourselves. A problem-solving strategy consists of how we perceive, store, and retrieve information about something. We initiate this problem-solving strategy by bringing the outside world inside us in order to interpret it. We do this through the use of our three predominant senses: visual (sight), auditory (hearing), and kinesthetic (bodily sensations, i.e., touch, muscle movements, etc.). To a much lesser degree we use our remaining two senses of taste and smell.

We then blend these external sensory stimuli with those we have stored inside of us called internal sensory stimuli. These internal resources include 1) pictures or images (visual); 2) self-talk (the auditory dialogue we constantly say to ourselves about what's going on); and 3) emotions (kinesthetic, internal body sensations).

Here is an example of the individual steps of the mindset process. You go to the fitness facility you've joined. You see two exercise classes going on simultaneously in rooms side by side (these classes are considered external visual stimuli), and hear the background music accompanying each class (external auditory stimuli). Both are using familiar exercise steps and gestures (external kinesthetic stimuli) you enjoy (enjoyment is an emotion which is an internally-felt kinesthetic stimuli). One workout session is a new activity you've never seen or done before, using a bench/step piece of equipment (you have no

visual/auditory/kinesthetic stimuli resources since you've never seen, heard, or felt it being used before). The other is a familiar aerobic dance-exercise class you've experienced many times before, (you have internal and external visual/auditory/kinesthetic resources present). The choice to join either session is yours, so which option do you choose?

Your problem-solving mechanism will be processing possible solutions to this question in split-seconds with your self-talk dialogue sounding similar to one of the following. Do you see, hear, and feel yourself in any of these particular solutions?

▶ "I enjoy the exercise-dance class (kinesthetic, emotions) and know the routines (kinesthetic, muscle movements). I just don't feel (kinesthetic, emotions) like thinking (processing new visual images, auditory sounds, and kinesthetic movements) and trying the new bench/step class right now." Or . . .

▶ "I feel so clumsy today (kinesthetic, both feelings and muscle movements), I know I'd slip (kinesthetic, muscle movements, and maybe visual pictures or auditory sounds) on the bench/step. I don't want or feel (kinesthetic, emotions) like having this new challenge (using all my senses to build resources) after the day I've had today!" Or . . .

▶ "Wow! I can do that (am willing to engage all three senses)! With a little direction (in developing new visual and auditory stimuli) on how and where to begin moving (kinesthetic, muscle movements), I'll have a new, fun, exciting choice to bring variety into my fitness-for-life program."

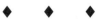

So, how you'll problem-solve the fitness choices you make (or ANY choices that you'll ever make, for that matter!), will come from your own internal thoughts, i.e., visual pictures you're making to yourself, auditory stimuli of external words and sounds or internal dialogue you're saying to yourself, and the kinesthetic stimuli or body sensations you're experiencing or choosing to experience.

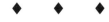

The lifestyle choices you make are, therefore, not made for you by someone or something else. *Your choices occur within you,* in that beautiful mental computer called your mind. . . ."Because thought results in behavior immediately, the only control that is ever needed is thought control, and that entails only my present willingness . . ."[1] The first step to understanding how to make healthy fitness choices is becoming aware of all of the resources that are available for us to use, both externally and internally.

You'll next recognize that external stimuli are available to all of us and that we all have the ability to create helpful internal stimuli that could lead to good choices. We must, however, *filter out* all the stimuli (both external and internal) that do not seem relevant at the moment to the problem at hand and focus only on what will fulfill our present, or most valued, wants or needs. (Again, this happens in fractions of seconds of time.) We complete this mindset process with a response, i.e., our *choice*!

So, how do we each uniquely filter through all of the multitude of sensory resources available to us and come up with poor or healthy choices? That key question is answered by understanding the remainder of the self-management model. Like dissecting layers of an apple and looking deeper within, we'll come to the center, the core, the programmed seed, understanding how we make the choices we do (Figure 1.2). Clarifying what directly precedes our choices is the next step in this looking-inward process.

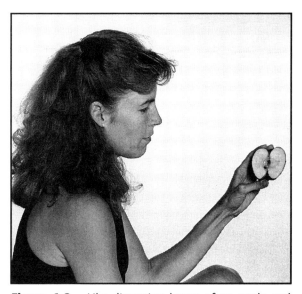

Figure 1.2. Like dissecting layers of an apple and looking deeper within, we'll come to the center, the core, the programmed seed, understanding how we make the choices we do.

THE EMOTIONAL FORCES THAT DIRECT AND CONTROL OUR CHOICES

We each have an innate survival mechanism within us that strongly encourages us to avoid pain and to gain pleasure. The dual forces of pain avoidance and

pleasure gratification are at work while we are problem-solving the challenges we face. For example, do we refuse the magnificent, high-calorie dessert our hostess has made especially for us at her home (emotional pain) and stick to our very firm commitment to ourselves to completely eliminate high-calorie/low nutrient desserts from our diet-intake? Or do we say "yes" (emotional pleasure), for whatever qualifying rationalized reasoning we come up with at the moment?

Problem-solving anything in our lives usually consists of trying to remove the problem (pain) as quickly as possible so that feeling good (pleasure) can again be ours on the forefront. We usually are quite unwilling to endure the emotional pain that all self-discipline, growth, and change seems to require. Another example we might say to ourselves, "Do I really have to do all these abdominal crunches every day (pain of waiting for the gratifying results) to have a tight, toned abdomen, or is there a short-cut (to the pleasure of having the results)? I hate strength training (pain, either emotional or physical). Maybe if I just don't eat as many sweets, my abdomen will get smaller, and look toned (instant pleasure gratification)."

The desire for pleasure is always the end result of *any* goal we have. Avoiding pain is viewed as the force we want to get rid of quickly, so we can experience the joy of feeling good (pleasure) once again (Figure 1.3). This may seem like common sense, but study what exactly is said here and all of

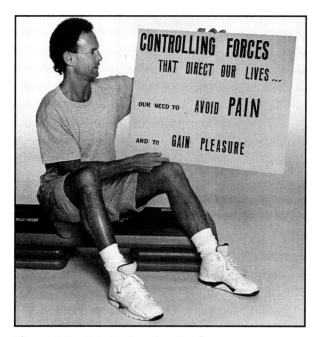

Figure 1.3. Pain is viewed as the force we want to get rid of quickly so we can experience the joy of feeling good.

the possible ramifications it could have on your ability to make healthful choices.

You will become aware that
another key to beginning and continuing
with a fitness commitment,
lies in your ability to learn to accept
the delaying of gratification
(delaying of pleasure, i.e., immediately having
the results you desire long-range),
and endure the growth and discipline
(endure the pain — the delaying of immediate
*   gratification)*
that is simply required for change —
permanently, blueprinted change   to occur.

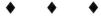

Mental techniques to assist you in achieving the delay of gratification in order to accommodate the time it takes to solidly blueprint a change of habits will be given later in the chapter and then again in Chapters 9 and 10. (The various emotions that make up the all-encompassing categories of pain and pleasure will be discussed more specifically in Chapter 9 to enable you to experience, in depth, the *re-linking* process that will occur when a fitness challenge perceived as painful becomes a pleasure.)

The next logical question: What determines whether we are directed and controlled by the force of pleasure and immediate gratification, or whether we can accept the pain of delaying instantly feeling good regarding the choices we make? We need to understand the third step inward in the self-management, mindset development process: What creates the willingness to endure waiting for growth and change to happen?

YOUR ATTITUDE

"The way we see things shapes the kinds of experiences we have . . . Our attitudes are truly the lenses of the mind through which we perceive reality . . . Up in your head and mine, are thousands of these attitudes . . . They are capable of making the same given experience either pleasant or painful." John Powell, SJ, Author.

Your attitude — that perspective or lens of positive and negative, open and closed-mindedness, and the enabling and disabling dispositions you take — are the true reflection of the opinion you have about something. When asked, most individuals will usually label themselves as having an overall positive attitude.

However, you only need to monitor your attitude for several days to realize how difficult it can be to maintain a positive outlook on life's many challenges.

Statistics from the medical and communication fields tell us that over 75% of all we experience is negative.[2] From the radio-TV-news media, to all the numerous other people we encounter, the volume of negative input we see, hear, and feel vastly outweighs the positive. So the challenge to remain firm in developing and keeping a positive, open mindset is tremendous. It takes a willingness and dedication on your part to actively and continuously choose it.

Choosing to establish, or keep, an open positive mindset as a lifestyle is made possible by becoming keenly aware of your attitude on problems and challenges experienced in your everyday living. One of the clearest reflections (i.e., easiest and most concrete means to experience if you are new at looking inward and observing how you perceive, store, and retrieve your information) is to listen and monitor — by writing down — your *self-talk*. Self-talk represents numerous ways to speak to yourself, out loud and silently within; and *about* yourself to others, out loud and in written and taped form.

We talk to ourselves 100% of our waking hours, about everything we're experiencing — seeing, hearing, emotionally feeling and physically touching, tasting and smelling. Taking a moment to observe your own self-talk and that of others, including media-talk, is the challenge presented to you to accept for the next several days. (See Charts 1, 2 and 3 in the Appendix.) It will be a real eye-opener, and the awareness you need to more quickly achieve some of the goals you'll soon set. "Mastery of communication is what makes a great [achiever]."[3]

In terms of making a change in your mindset, you'll observe that negative self-talk is said or recorded using past and future tense verbs. Positive self-talk is stated and recorded in the present tense, and/or uses verbs ending in *ing*, creating the feeling that the present action is happening now.

In addition to your self-talk, a second clear indicator of your attitude is experienced through your kinesthetic sense — *your physiologies and how you move*. For example, "when exercising . . . if you work hard and you're short of breath and you keep saying to yourself how tired you are or how far you've run, you will indulge in a physiology-like panting or sitting down — that supports that communication. If, however, even though you're out of breath — you consciously stand upright and direct your breathing into a normal rate, you will feel recovered in a matter of moments."[4]

A third indicator of your attitude may at first be rather abstract to experience or "see" for the novice, but with awareness and practice it can be as powerful as your self-talk and physiological expressions. It involves the *mental images or pictures you make* and, how close/far away, color/black-and-white, moving/still, etc., they are, and whether you are in the images (associated), or removed from the images and are observing (disassociated). There is a vast amount of exciting research going on concerning all three of these factors that influence attitude, and one's health and fitness. The body of information called neuro-linguistic programming or NLP, and the relatively new science of psychoneuroimmunology are both good resources to look into, if you desire more information on the topic.[5]

"Studies in neuroscience and psychobiology have shown that the way you think can affect your body and its performance. For example, stressful events perceived as threatening produce hormones in the body that reduce exercise efficiency and increase fatigue. However, when a stressful situation is viewed in a more positive light, as a challenge rather than a threat, other chemicals . . . are released in the body producing improved exercise performance."[6]

Once you are aware of how powerfully the factors that make up your attitude affect your adherence to a fitness program, it will become an exciting challenge to do something constructive to improve them to bring about the changes you desire. It will be very motivating to develop repetitive, positive self-talk (called *affirmations*), enabling physiologies (more effective postures and breathing techniques), and positive images (which are more colorful, closeup, and active) that you're now choosing to hear, feel, and see about yourself and your program. (Programming techniques are in Chapters 1, 9, and 10.) "If you are consistently delivering congruent messages to your nervous system that say you *can* do something, they signal your brain to produce the result you desire, and that opens up the possibility for it."[7]

So, the key thought with attitudes is openness — saying, picturing, and feeling "I can!" and then remaining open for the answer to *how.* Your brain will continually search for possibilities when the channels and pathways are kept open.

Clearly, your attitude is a key to having a mindset for successful, healthy living. But, you'll immediately become aware that just *telling* yourself positive affirmation statements, or *visualizing* helpful images, or engaging in various *motivational* movements regarding goals you'd like to achieve (and actually *achieving* the goals) can be two separate phenomena — if your search for solutions stops there. But it doesn't.

What does determine your ability to color an experience or perspective positively or negatively? What is responsible for developing your attitudes and cementing them permanently, for adherence and

consistency? It's time to go one step deeper within, and take a look at *what lies at the foundation of the entire mindset process.* What seed lies at the core of our choices?

YOUR BELIEFS: THE KEY TO UNDERSTANDING YOUR PROGRAMMING

Whether you call them guiding principles, rules for living, faith, philosophies for life, or truths you value, your beliefs ultimately determine the behavioral choices you make. Some of the beliefs we hold originated out of an intensely significant experience (one where all of our senses were *vividly* involved) and some, over time, by a collection of less intense experiences. So what are beliefs? Here are a few definitions to ponder:

▶ useful thoughts that can provide meaning and direction in life;

▶ statements that we have accepted as the truth and are useful, and have been given to us by all the significant people in our life that we trust: parents, grandparents, pastors/rabbis/priests, relatives, brothers and sisters, peers, teachers, coaches, advisors, specific media sources, etc.;

▶ pre-arranged, organized filters to our perceptions of the world;

▶ commanders of the brain, which deliver a direct command to our nervous system;

▶ the *compass* and *maps* that guide us toward our goals.

What is remarkable is that we continually make choices based on the programmed beliefs we have and value, and many times these beliefs are old, worn out hand-me-downs that we've just accepted and never really questioned for personal validity. Since you are now in a maturing process within your life's journey, where intellectual growth is expected along with physical development, be sure the beliefs you are following concerning fitness and developing a healthy mindset are the best around! There is no universal rule that states that old worn out programmed beliefs can't be changed. Life *is* change and growth and involves the stretching of one's self to the limits of his or her own potential.

Have you ever pondered the fact that the people who have significantly changed history have been the people who have greatly changed our beliefs? Stop for a moment and think about that; then realize that your beliefs can really help you to change an unwanted behavior, especially if you have some key new beliefs that work, are useful, and do not infringe upon the wants and needs of others.

Begin to more closely observe behavior, emotions, attitudes, and beliefs of present-day people who are successful role models of excellence and who exemplify the fitness lifestyle you'd like to have. Their positive strategies may contribute to your success.

Take a moment now and begin to establish a collection of beliefs you have about living a healthy lifestyle. Chart 4 in the Appendix is provided to get you started. Several samples of enabling beliefs, taken from the master role models of our time, are included. If you like them, they're yours to adopt, too. Continue listing enabling helpful beliefs as you continue through your fitness course. Stating, picturing, and feeling yourself believing these thoughts will assist you with blueprinting the fitness for-life mindset.

One exciting way to more readily accomplish this permanent blueprinting process is by constructing your own programmed audiotape. Using your information identified on Charts 1 through 4 in the Appendix, and following the procedures concerning making your own self-management tape on Chart 5 in the Appendix, you'll have a very powerful tool to help you to change and experience new results in about three weeks!

♦   ♦   ♦

New Beginnings

By doing what needs to be done right now,
we make the most of each present moment.
As long as we are alive,
we are always free to begin again.
Instead of following an old, worn-out habit,
make a fresh start this moment
on the rest of your life.
Each day is a new start.
Each moment is a beginning. (Anon.)

♦   ♦   ♦

SUMMARY

The process of developing a mindset for the fitness lifestyle includes becoming more aware of 1) the choices we constantly make, and 2) what internal resources we've used to make these choices.

Choices we make can be experienced by us and others. We can clearly see, hear, and feel these responses. What we can't immediately detect is *how* — what process — led us to that conclusion. Taking the process apart, step by step, helps us to know where our mindset needs repair and allows us to insert new constructive possibilities. Immediately preceding or underlying our choices, then, are our emotions, attitudes, and beliefs. Our beliefs are our ultimate valued guidelines for living that we have fully accepted and allowed to become programmed onto our own mental tapes. *So if we are to change our choices, we must ultimately update our disabling, no longer useful, beliefs.*

Change is a choice.

Chapter 2

The Fitness Lifestyle — Physically Achieved Through Aerobic Exercise

COMBINING MENTAL CONDITIONING WITH PHYSICAL FITNESS

Consider for a moment now, these two very familiar philosophies we often hear: "Use it or lose it!" and "Knowledge is power!" Do you ever quote either of these? Or perhaps, both? Both are quite brief, yet very powerful beliefs that can actually put to the test the mindset for the fitness lifestyle you are now developing.

The first belief — "Use it or lose it!" — is one that can be applied to all the dimensions of your physical wellness and one that must rank at the very top of the priority list of choices when it comes to achieving and maintaining a physically healthy lifestyle. The second belief — "Knowledge is power!" — sounds good, but actually is in need of the updating before it can become a belief that is actually working for us. Knowledge of all the fitness benefits, or test results will not be enough to change a sedentary mindset or improve one's total physical fitness. *Actions* must be combined with all this knowledge. Updating the latter belief to read, "The application of knowledge is power!" is a completed thought and will enable us to get moving!

Get Motivated!

The opening message to begin the journey of understanding how to obtain physical fitness through participation in an activity like aerobics (dance-exercise) is therefore pretty simple: Don't just sit back and absorb and do nothing with all the wealth of unique and fantastic ideas coming your way through this text and course! Think creatively: "How can I use each point of knowledge as it comes to me?" *By immediately developing powerful images, internal self-talk, and emotion-filled movements regarding the information it will help you to retain it, to solidly "blueprint" it, so that other information can be systematically built upon it later.*

~ These 3 key elements ~

▶ *powerful images,*

▶ *internal self-talk,*

▶ *emotion-filled movements*

are the basic building blocks of the abstract thought we call *MOTIVATION!*

Get Ready — Get Set — For The Researched Findings

Our mental approach to the physical fitness challenge has been established. We are armed with how to become motivated and we arc *ready*! It's time to *set* the stage and solidify, with reasons, facts, statistics, etc., why one should go-for-it-all and become physically fit.

Physical conditioning through an activity like aerobics will assure you a happier, more vivacious, and abundant life. Or, stated in even more dramatic terms, the physically fit active lifestyle prolongs life![1]

"We've moved beyond fantasy, to the reality that cardiovascular fitness can indeed reduce the risks of killer diseases and enhance the prospects for a longer, more energetic life."[2] "The number of adults exercising 20 minutes three times a week jumped from only 28% in 1968 to 59% in 1984. During the same time, deaths from heart disease dropped 48% and life expectancy has risen five years to about [age] 75."[3] Furthermore, "Some predictions are that by the end of this century, the average American woman will live to age ninety, and the average American man to the mid-eighties."[4] With these impressive findings and a projected long life ahead of us, let's make sure it will be a *quality* long life we're living (not just doing time), by making good choices.

Aerobic/Aerobics/Aerobic Dance-Exercise

Within the research just quoted, the key word *aerobic* was introduced and tied to the active life-style. Just what does this term mean?

Most simply stated, the term aerobic is an adjective which means *promoting the supply and use of oxygen*. The body's demand for oxygen will increase when you engage in vigorous activity that produces specific beneficial changes in the body. Aerobic can, therefore, refer to *any type of exercise mode as long as certain basic criteria are met*.

Take note, however, that within the last decade, the exercise mode originally entitled *aerobic dance*, then more generalized to the term *aerobic exercise* has been shortened simply for brevity to the currently popular terms aerobics or aerobic dance-exercise. These two terms (aerobics and aerobic dance-exercise) now replace formerly used terminology and are interchangeably used to mean the same activity throughout this text, as it is throughout the professional journals of today. Therefore, keep a clear distinction: aerobic is used as an adjective describing another word, and *aerobics* is used as a noun: a mode of activity.

Healthy Life-Style Choices

Associated regular fitness behaviors that enhance your ability to perform well during your physical conditioning workout include: eating nutritionally, maintaining a proper body weight, relaxing, and getting an adequate amount of sleep. Without a balance in your *biochemical functioning*, i.e., your energy intake, energy expenditure, and energy rejuvenation, the effects and benefits mentioned later will not occur. Several highlights concerning each of these healthy life-style choices follow. A complete chapter of information on each is presented later in the text.

Eating

In order to provide the fuel needed to produce the energy required for all aerobic exercise, and to insure proper body regulatory functions, growth, and repair, eat a well-balanced diet that provides all the nutrients you need to stay well, to be able to perform well, and to maintain a proper weight.

Regarding how much to eat and the time of day for eating, it is suggested that food intake involve a 25–50–25 rule, i.e., 25% of intake for breakfast, 50% for lunch, and 25% for supper. Incidentally, you'll find that weight control is easier for those who either exercise before breakfast, or one and one-half hours after the heaviest meal of the day.[5]

Other guidelines regarding when to eat in relation to your exercise program are the following. For greatest efficiency, refrain from eating for one, or preferably two, hours before participating in aerobic activity. *Eat afterward*. With the digestion of food, an increased amount of blood and oxygen is needed in the digestive tract. With exercise, as much as 100 times more oxygen is needed in the working muscles, i.e., arms and legs, than when at rest. Your body will have great difficulty supplying an increase in blood and oxygen to two major body functions at once!

Relaxing and Sleeping

Establish quality time for reflective relaxation, and adequate sleep. These are important restorative mechanisms in several ways. Since aerobics will expend a great deal of energy, the body's way of restoring energy is through relaxation and sleep. Each helps to restore the ability to concentrate and to maintain a positive attitude.

Physiologically, relaxation and sleep help by lowering both the body temperature and heart rate, which, in turn, lower the body's demand for oxygen and nutrients. These, therefore, conserve while restoring the body's supply of energy.

A Total Physical Fitness Conditioning Program

Total physical fitness is that positive state of well-being in which you have enough strength and energy to participate in a full active lifestyle of your own choice. It's "the general capacity to adapt favorably to physical effort. An individual is physically fit when s/he is able to meet both the usual and unusual demands of daily life, safely and effectively without undue stress or exhaustion." (American Medical Association)

A total physical fitness conditioning program consists of five basic parts and can be visualized by the fitness triangle, depicting three action-type components, centered around two underlying structural components (Figure 2.1).

1. **Aerobic Fitness** (cardiovascular and respiratory)

2. **Flexibility** (ability to bend and stretch)

3. **Muscular Strength and Muscular Endurance** (thickening muscle fiber mass to enable individuals to endure a heavier work load)

4. **Good Posture** (body always held in proper positioning for safety and efficiency)

5. **Body Composition** (maintaining proper fat weight to lean weight ratio).

Aerobic Fitness

A total, well-rounded weekly fitness conditioning program should consist of attention to and regular participation in all five components. However, since the sign of genuine fitness is the condition of your heart, your blood vessels, and your lungs, aerobic fitness is the most important component. By engaging in aerobic dance-exercise, or any other aerobic activity (like the currently very popular step-training) your heart gradually strengthens and develops a greater capacity to pump more oxygenated blood to the body with fewer contractions (exercised hearts are stronger and slower).

"Highly trained and conditioned endurance athletes have resting heart rates as low as 30 to 32 beats per minute, an unbelievably low rate! What actually happens is that with regular, stimulating exercise, the heart becomes a more efficient pump. It pumps more blood with each stroke, and with a more efficient stroke volume, your heart can function with less effort. By getting your heart into condition, you may be practicing preventive medicine. You may be lessening the danger of a coronary heart attack, five, ten, fifteen, twenty years from now. And if you do have one, your chances of surviving are far greater with a heart, and lungs, and blood vessels which are in good condition."[6]

It is thought-provoking to realize that you can still exist without big bulging muscles, or without the perfect figure, or with a head cold, but that you can't exist very long without a good heart and lungs. Unfortunately, more than 40 percent of all people who have their first heart attack do not receive a second chance to change their habits, or develop an aerobic program — they die.[7] And over one-half of all American deaths last year were due to heart-related diseases.[8] If only we could establish a living pattern priority early in life to correct this overwhelming statistic.

Flexibility

This second physical fitness component is the functional range of motion of a certain joint and its corresponding muscle groups. The greater the range of movement, the more the muscles, tendons, and ligaments can flex or bend. Muscles are arranged in pairs. One muscle's ability to shorten or contract is directly related to the opposing muscle's length or stretch. Flexibility is maintained or increased by movement patterns that slowly and progressively stretch the muscle beyond its relaxed length. The stretch is performed to a point where tension developing in the muscle is felt, but not to a point of pain.

Muscular Strength and Muscular Endurance

Muscular strength is the ability of a muscle to exert a force against a resistance. Strength activities increase the amount of force that muscles can exert, or the amount of work that muscles can perform. Activities such as weight training can develop strength in the skeletal muscles.

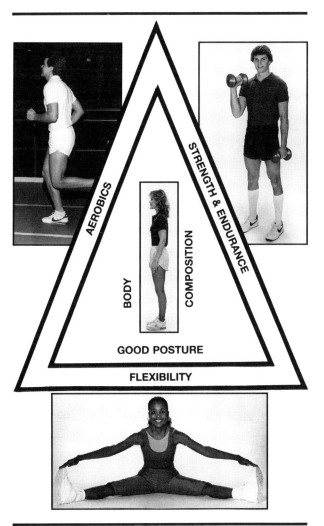

Figure 2.1. Fitness triangle.

Muscular endurance is the ability of muscles to work strenuously for progressively longer periods of time without fatigue. It is the capacity of a muscle to exert a force repeatedly, or to hold a static (still) contraction over a period of time.

Muscular strength and endurance activities do not provide a vigorous increased usage of oxygen to condition the heart to function more efficiently[9]; their primary target is skeletal muscle.

Good Posture (i.e., Good Positioning)

Proper positioning of the body when performing any type of physical exertion will insure a safe and efficient workout. Once the basic mechanics are known and practiced, this underlying fitness component is performed as an integral part of every move you make, and not as a separate program of its own.

Body Composition

An individual's total body weight is comprised of fat weight and lean weight (fat-free weight). Keeping an appropriate percentage ratio between these two weights is important for your entire system's best functioning, and to help in preventing the onset of obesity and its many related health risks. As with the good posture component of the total physical fitness picture, there is no *separate* physical fitness program in which to engage for the body composition component. *By establishing a proper diet and exercise plan that provides for ideal weight maintenance, this fitness component is managed.*

There will be very specific guidelines given within both the physical exercise programs and the dietary eating plans you'll establish, for how to achieve your ideal percentage ratio, if you aren't beginning your program at your ideal weight.

In summation, the five components to consider when developing a total physical fitness conditioning workout program (i.e., your *prescription exercise plan*) are: aerobic (cardiorespiratory) fitness training; flexibility training; muscular strength and endurance training; good posture; and maintaining proper body composition, for your entire system's best functioning.

Since aerobic fitness training is considered the most important component of these five, the remainder of Chapter 2 will be devoted to a detailed look at the research and general principles that are recommended for you to follow, including modes of activity you choose and the individual techniques you use. The other four physical fitness components are explained in depth later in other chapters.

AEROBIC FITNESS TRAINING

Aerobic Capacity Improvement — Your Main Objective

Since aerobic means promoting the supply and use of oxygen, and training refers to muscle stimulation, aerobic exercise is any exercise which requires a steady supply of oxygen for an extended time period and demands an uninterrupted work output from your muscles.

Activities like aerobic dance-exercise and step-training significantly increase the oxygen supply to all body parts, including the heart and lungs, through continuous, rhythmic movement of large muscles and connective tissue. This type of movement conditions the body's oxygen transport system (the heart, lungs, blood, and blood vessels) to process the use of oxygen more efficiently. This *efficiency in processing oxygen* is called your *aerobic capacity* and is dependent on your ability to:

▶ Rapidly breathe large amounts of air.

▶ Forcefully deliver large volumes of blood.

▶ Effectively deliver oxygen to all parts of the body.

In short, your aerobic capacity depends upon efficient lungs, a powerful heart, and a good vascular system. Because it reflects the conditions of these vital organs, *the aerobic capacity is the best index (single measure) of overall physical fitness.*[10]

Aerobic capacity is what is measured, quantified, and labeled in a physical fitness stress test, performed either in a laboratory (called a laboratory stress test) or on a pre-measured distance like a track (called a field stress test). You are given the opportunity to test your aerobic capacity in Chapter 3, using either method.

Strengthening The Heart: Progressive Overload Principle

Aerobic dance-exercise, step-training, or any aerobic activity, conditions the heart muscle by strengthening it through a principle called *progressive overload*. Not only will the heart pump more blood with each beat, it will have longer rests between each beat, therefore lowering the pulse rate. Aerobic exercise overloads the heart by simply causing it to beat faster during a specific time-frame of the workout session, making a temporary high demand on the cardiorespiratory system. Over time, as you become more fit, the heart eventually adjusts to this temporary high demand and soon it is able to do the same amount of work with less effort.

Your goal is to achieve the training effect. By *overloading* the heart with any vigorous aerobic exercise, your aerobic capacity is increased and a desirable training effect can be achieved. The *training effect*, or total beneficial changes that usually occur are:

▶ Stronger heart sending more oxygenated blood to all tissues of the body.

▶ More blood cells produced.

▶ Slower resting heart rate.

▶ Expansion of blood vessels.

▶ Improvement of muscle tone.

▶ A lowering of blood pressure through improved circulation.

▶ Stronger respiratory muscles.

▶ Regulates the release of adrenalin.

▶ Increased lung capacity.

▶ A more regular elimination of solid wastes.

▶ Lower levels of fat found in blood.[11]

▶ Strengthens muscles and skeleton to protect them from injury later in life.

▶ By increasing bone density, it helps prevent osteoporosis.[12]

▶ Increased sensitivity to insulin and lowered blood sugar levels in mild, adult-onset diabetes.[13]

▶ Improves the way cholesterol is handled by the body, by increasing the proportion of blood cholesterol attached to high-density lipoprotein — a carrier molecule that keeps cholesterol from damaging artery walls.[14]

AEROBIC EXERCISE ALTERNATIVES

Aerobic exercise options include all of the following activities. Principles and program techniques that are presented in this text are in bold type.

▶ **Aerobic Dance-Exercise** (i.e., **Aerobics**).

▶ **Bench / Step-Training.**

▶ Cross-Country Skiing.

▶ Cycling (including Stationary Cycling).

▶ **Jogging / Running.**

▶ **Jumping Rope**.

▶ Rowing.

▶ Skating (Ice/Roller/Roller Blade).

▶ Stair Climbing.

▶ Swimming.

▶ **Walking**/Hiking (moderate to fast pace-walk).

Aerobic Criteria

Each of these exercise alternatives, collectively, have several essential criteria that must be present, however, in order for the exercise to be labeled *aerobic* (see Figure 2.2). Since *aerobic* means *with oxygen*, the movement that you do must:

1. **Use the large muscles of the body,**[15] i.e., your arms and legs. Exercise gesture and step patterns found in aerobic dance-exercise and bench-step movements are excellent choices!

2. **Be rhythmic,**[16] one-two-one-two, using a steady beat of music, with either a fast or slow tempo.

3. **Practice for a minimum of three sessions per week.**[17]

   ▶ Four days a week or every other day is good.

   ▶ Some key researchers state five days is a maximum for fitness goals. Beyond this, injuries are ten times more likely to occur to the musculoskeletal system from overuse. So, give your body at least two days off per week, especially if you are a novice to physical fitness conditioning.

   ▶ If your goals are more than just aerobic fitness related — if perhaps your profession (like fitness instructor) or your athletic sport-status requires more workouts or days per week, allow your body to *tell you* your maximum frequency. A sudden elevated resting heart rate in the morning will be the day(s) not to workout. This is your built in body signal and it can be readily seen/heard/felt simply by daily monitoring your resting heart rate. Check this heart rate for one full minute upon arising in the morning.

4. **Exercise continuously for a time duration of 20–60 minutes.**[18]

   ▶ Duration is dependent upon the *intensity* and *impact* of the activity. (Both of these terms are explained later in full detail.)

   ▶ Lower intensity activity, such as walking, should be conducted over a longer period of time i.e., 40–60 minutes.

   ▶ Because high impact types of activity, such as running and jumping, generally cause significantly more debilitating injuries to exercisers, the shorter workout (20 minutes) is recommended.

5. And, in order to receive the cardiorespiratory fitness benefits (called the training effect), **the heart rate must be maintained in a specific**

FIT =

INTENSITY

FREQUENCY

Sun.	Mon.	Tues.	Wed.	Thur.	Fri.	Sat.
	1	2	3	4	5	6
7	8	9	10	11	12	13
14	15	16	17	18	19	20
21	22	23	24	25	26	27
28	29	30	31			

- **At least 3 times per week.**
- **Every other day is best.**
- **Maximum of 5 days per week.**

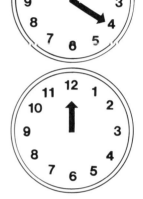

- **65-90%* of maximal heart rate or 50-85%* of VO2 max; according to your fitness level.**
- **And, use large muscles & be rhythmic.**

TIME

- **20 minutes to 60 minutes* duration of time recommended, according to intensity and impact.**
- **30 minutes for most activities.**

Figure 2.2. Five aerobic criteria.

target heart rate training zone, which is the individualized safe pace at which to aerobically work or exercise. This reflects your intensity and is scientifically explained as one of the following:

▶ 65–90 percent of your maximum heart rate; or

▶ 50–85 percent of your maximum oxygen uptake, or heart rate reserve.[19]

Intensity Detailed

Frequency and time duration of your workouts are easy to determine. However, how much exertion you perform during the workout to keep it safe and continually making fitness gains can be a little bit more of a challenge to determine, especially for the novice.

Intensity is measured or monitored in one of three ways:

▶ Finding your *target heart rate training zone* (THR) using the Karvonen formula is suggested for the novice.

▶ Using the psychophysical scale for *ratings of perceived exertion* (RPE) which shows a high correlation with heart rate and other metabolic parameters according to American College Sports Medicine guidelines. Rate of perceived exertion monitoring is suggested for the individual who has already become well-accustomed to taking a heart rate pulse.

▶ The *Talk Test*. This easy and practical method is best used when in conjunction with the THR and RPE for monitoring exercise intensity.

Your Target Heart Rate Training Zone

Taking Your Pulse

To calculate appropriate exercise intensity using this method, you first must know how to accurately take your pulse. The pulse equals heartbeats per minute and can be felt and counted in one of six pulsation points. Select at which area you can best obtain a pulse, using your index and second fingers. The two places most often used for pulse counting are on the neck near the carotid artery, and on the wrist near the radial artery.

1. The carotid artery is located in the neck and is usually easy to find (see Figure 2.3). Place your index and middle fingers *below the point of your jawbone* and slide downward an inch or so, pressing lightly, When you use the carotid artery pulse-monitoring method, make sure that you apply light pressure, as excessive pressure may cause the heart rate to slow down by a reflex action.

2 The radial artery extends up the wrist on the thumb side (see Figure 2.4). Place your index and middle fingers just below the base of your thumb. Press lightly. Now count the number of

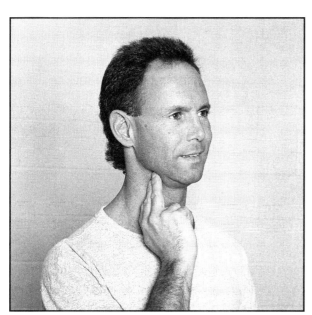

Figure 2.3. Taking the carotid pulse.

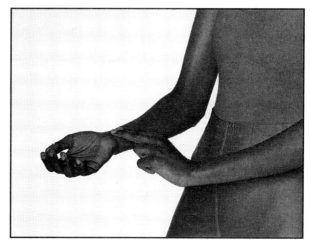

Figure 2.4. Taking the radial pulse.

pulsations, or beats, for 60 seconds. The total is the number of heartbeats per minute. To count correctly, make sure that you count each beat you feel.

Having gained the skill of pulse taking, it is now time to establish your *resting heart rate*. This figure needs to be placed in the formula for establishing your target heart rate training zone.

Monitoring the Resting Pulse Rate

A true *resting heart rate* (RsHR) is not taken in a class but when the individual has been at complete rest (i.e., sleeping) for several hours and just awakens. Keep a clock or watch with a second hand next to your bed. When you awaken (without an alarm clock ring), take your pulse for one full minute and record that number as your RsHR on Chart 6 in the Appendix. Do this for five consecutive mornings, then determine an average (add all RsHR's and divide by five). This is a rather accurate determination of your resting heart rate.

Note

Unusual stress and illness (illness is a type of stress) will sharply elevate the resting heart rate from previous readings.

You will understand why it is so important, then, for normally healthy individuals to find a positive outlet for stress; it affects you even as you sleep (constant rapid heart rate), a time when the heart ideally should take a break and slow down for six to eight hours.

Continue to record your RsHR twice a week thereafter until the conclusion of the eight-to-ten-week course. Record your final reading after your initial reading and determine the loss or gain in RsHR for the eight-to-ten-week period.

One of the two visible signs of improvement in heart and lung fitness that you will experience is a lowering of the resting heart rate. Because the RsHR is the basic thermometer of fitness, after a ten-to-fifteen-week aerobics course you and your classmates may experience similar results:

▶ An average –3 heartbeats per minute resting heart rate decline.

▶ An average –10 heartbeats per minute recorded by smokers who quit (or significantly change their consumption) during the course, with as much as a –24 heartbeats per minute decline recorded. [20]

Determining Your Target Heart Rate Training Zone

Your average RsHR figure is now placed in the formula for determining your target heart rate training zone, as found on Chart 7 in the Appendix. The other variables that are figured into the formula are your current *age* and your *lifestyle*, represented as a percentage of your maximum heart rate.

IF YOU ARE:	USE:
▶ a non-athletic adult	50% to begin
▶ sedentary	60–69%
▶ moderately active	70–75%
▶ very active and well-trained	80–85%

Place your age and the selected percentage range from above that describes your lifestyle. Figure the Karvonen equation: the result is your target heart rate, the safe exercise training zone for you.

Immediate Count Taken After An Aerobics Interval

As you are beginning an aerobics program, you'll want to monitor your pace several times during the workout hour so that you can develop the skill of constant endurance pacing. Mentally remember your readings and record them at the end of class. Chart 8 in the Appendix is provided for this monitoring.

When you take a pulse rate during the learning process and find that your pace is *below* your established training zone, increase your intensity. If you are experiencing a pulse rate *higher* than your established training zone, lower your intensity.

In order to become familiar with your own response to various intensity levels so that you can better regulate yourself, ask yourself, *"How do I feel when I get this pulse?"* Remember, focus not only on your pulse count, but on what feelings and conditions the number relates to, so that you can develop recognition of the signals your body gives. This will also assist you in developing skills to use the RPE

monitoring method of intensity, which as you become a more advanced exerciser, will be the more practical and practiced method you'll probably use, instead of counting your heart rate beats per minute.

Continuing at a pace that is too intense will prove to be an *anaerobic* exercise program. *Anaerobic* activity is basically activity that is stop and start, or one in which the heart is not kept at a constant steady pace for twenty to sixty minutes. Thus, anaerobic describes an activity that requires an all-out effort of short duration and that does not utilize oxygen to produce energy. This type of exercise quickly uses up more oxygen than the body can take in while engaging in the exercise, causing an oxygen debt. This, in turn, causes lactic acids (waste products) to accumulate in the muscles, which leads to exhaustion.

The pulse-monitoring procedure during aerobics is then to slow down, walk around, find your pulse, and count it for either six or ten seconds. Each of these counts has been found to be a scientifically accurate measurement for aerobic activity pulse rates. Taking the immediate count after aerobic exercise using a timed count of greater than ten seconds will tend to be inaccurate, since the heart rate slows down to a *recovery* pulse rather rapidly. You or your instructor will determine whether you will count for six or ten seconds. Immediately following the aerobic exercise segment, count your pulse and multiply the number you get times ten if using the six-second count, or times six if using a ten-second count. Each of these newly multiplied numbers will equal heartbeats per minute and hopefully will always be in your training zone.

Note

It is easy to take a six-second count; all you do is add a zero to what pulse you feel and record that number. You must carefully begin and end exactly with a timer.

Table 2.1 lists target heart rate counts for individuals who wish to attain fitness using the ideal aerobic range for most people, i.e., 60–75% of heart rate reserve. Locate the column across the top that is closest to your age and the row down the left side reflecting a figure closest to your resting heart rate. The box where the column and row intersect is *your ten second target heart rate training zone.*

Also you will soon recognize that, as your cardio-respiratory system becomes more fit and efficient, work (exercise) will become easier, and you will be forced to increase the intensity of your activities. Techniques for increasing and decreasing the intensity of your workout will be fully explained in Chapter 4. By using the target heart rate training zone, you automatically compensate for increased

TABLE 2.1   **Target Heart Rate Training Zones***

Your Age ▶

Your Av. Resting Heart Rate ▼	15	20	25	30	35	40	45	50	55	60	65	70	75	80
90	27-29	26-29	26-28	25-28	25-27	24-26	23-26	23-25	22-24	22-24	21-23	21-22	20-22	20-21
85	26-29	26-29	25-28	25-27	24-27	24-26	23-25	23-25	22-24	22-24	21-23	21-22	20-22	20-21
80	26-29	25-28	25-28	24-27	24-26	23-26	23-25	22-25	22-24	21-23	21-23	20-22	20-21	19-21
75	26-29	25-28	25-28	24-27	24-26	23-26	23-25	22-25	21-24	21-23	20-23	20-22	19-21	19-21
70	25-29	25-28	24-27	24-27	23-26	23-25	22-25	22-24	21-24	21-24	20-22	20-22	19-21	19-20
65	25-28	25-28	24-27	23-26	23-26	22-25	21-24	21-24	21-23	20-23	20-22	19-21	19-21	18-20
60	25-28	24-28	24-27	23-26	23-26	22-25	21-24	21-24	20-23	20-22	19-22	19-21	18-21	18-20
55	24-27	23-27	23-27	23-26	22-25	21-24	21-24	21-24	20-23	20-22	19-22	19-21	18-20	18-20
50	24-28	23-27	23-26	22-26	22-25	21-25	21-24	20-23	20-23	19-22	19-21	18-21	18-20	17-20

*The numbers in the squares represent pulse beats counted in ten seconds.

fitness and still maintain the same training effect. Thus, your heart rate will increase during vigorous aerobic activity and should, likewise, return to normal (normal meaning a pre-activity heart rate) within a short period of time after the workout. As a rule, the faster it slows down (i.e., recovers from exercise), the more physically fit you are, for recovery heart rate improvement is another indication of an increased fitness level!

The Borg Scale: Ratings of Perceived Exertion

The second method for monitoring your intensity is using the psychophysical Borg scale for ratings of perceived exertion (RPE)[21], as shown in Table 2.2. This scale is based on the finding that while exercising, one has the ability to accurately assess how hard their body is working. It's basically a judgment call and is "more appropriate when used by individuals who have been exercising for a while." The untrained exerciser typically reports a higher RPE than an athlete at the same exercise heart rate.

RPE seems to correlate strongly with other workload indicators, such as ventilation, oxygen consumption, and muscle metabolism. Participants tune into the overall sensation of effort exerted by their entire body, rather than one factor such as local calf or hamstring exhaustion, panting, sweating, or body temperature. RPE, when used along with heart rate monitoring, is very useful for the novice, who may not yet be aware of how exercise is supposed to feel.

You are invited to begin to make mental notes to yourself during the workout hour concerning your ratings of perceived exertion. After the workout is over, immediately record what you felt for each phase of the workout, expressed as numbers from 0–10. Chart 8, Side B in the Appendix is provided for this recording. Begin to notice the correlation between target heart rates achieved and how ratings of perceived exertion feel.

The Talk Test

There is a third and less formal method for determining aerobic intensity called the *talk test*. It is based on the premise that, while exercising, the participant should always be able to hold a conversation. If the participant can only gasp out one or two words at a time, the exercise intensity is probably anaerobic and should be adjusted to allow for two- to three-word phrases. Since the accuracy of the talk test varies within any given population, it is, therefore, best utilized in conjunction with the THR and the RPE for monitoring exercise intensity.[28]

TABLE 2.2   Borg Scale Ratings of Perceived Exertion[21]

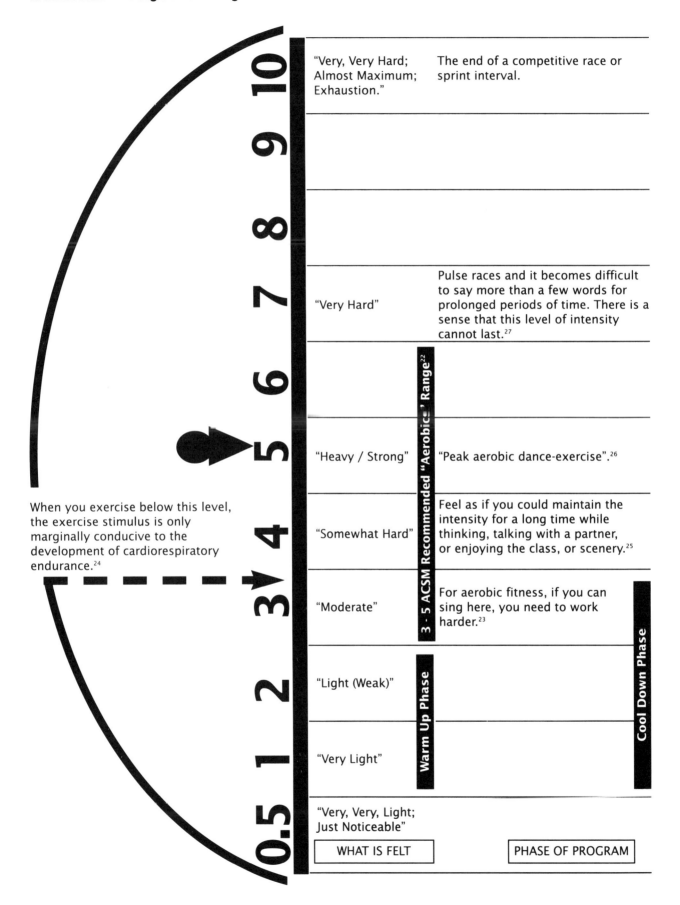

Which Method Is Best?

The experts do not agree when it comes to THR vs. RPE. Some claim that only THR methods are accurate; others believe that RPE and the talk test are more practical. Since all the methods are useful and none is consistently ideal, a good solution to the question of "Which method should I use?" is this: *use a combination of all three!* Once a participant has developed a good understanding of the heart rate/RPE relationship, heart rate can be monitored less frequently and RPE can be used as a primary means of measuring exercise intensity with the talk test as an informal supplemental backup measure.[29]

IMPACT: HIGH, LOW, COMBINATION HIGH/LOW, & MODERATE

There is one more ingredient in the aerobics formula for fitness to consider when establishing your prescription for exercise, of how often (frequency), how much work (heart rate beats per minute/intensity), and how long to work out (duration of time per session). This is the concept of impact that needs to be included when determining the time duration you spend per session of aerobic exercise.

Basic step movements in aerobics have experienced much change since the origin of the activity. These changes have centered around injury reduction and prevention, with the primary focus centered on the amount of vertical force exerted on the feet as they contact (impact) with the floor surface and how this stress subsequently effects the musculoskeletal system.

Early programs included many steps and gestures with great bodily elevation and with a likewise great compression when foot contact was made with the floor. Research has given the aerobics enthusiast a variety of safe alternatives when it comes to impact and movement possibilities.

IMPACT EVALUATION

High-Impact Aerobics (HIA)

This style of impact involves steps and gestures in which there is a brief moment when both feet may be off the floor at the same time. This step and gesture movement selection results in a great force being exerted when the foot meets the floor surface. This force will be absorbed by the landing, floor surface, shoes, orthotics (if worn), and the musculoskeletal system (muscles, tendons, ligaments, joints and bones).

Several examples of basic movements that are considered high-impact are jogging, hopping, and jumping. Below are a few characteristics of high-impact aerobics:

▶ Music between 130–160 BPM's.
▶ Faster music, smaller moves.
▶ Slower music, greater range of motion.
▶ Land through toe/ball/heel.
▶ Avoid over 8 reps on one limb.
▶ Strengthen anterior tibialis (shin area).
▶ Strengthen hamstrings.
▶ Limit to every other day.
▶ Higher intensity = > VO$_2$ max.
▶ Moderate intensity = > fat utilization.[30]

And, high-impact aerobics (HIA) is generally *not recommended* for the following:

▶ Individuals who are obviously deconditioned or out of shape, especially if they are obese.
▶ Anyone who is susceptible to specific injuries (such as shin splints) that are caused by, or likely to be aggravated by, upward impacts on the feet.
▶ Women in the latter stages of pregnancy who usually have loosening of the joints.
▶ Individuals who suffer from incontinence.
▶ Participants who are simply uncomfortable with high-impact steps.[31]

Low-Impact Aerobics (LIA)

This impact style involves steps and gestures that will cause less force when the foot strikes the floor than those found in traditional impact movements. Great control over the landing and force of foot impact is present, since there is one foot kept in contact with the floor at all times.

Take note, however. *Low-impact does not mean low-intensity!* Cardiorespiratory conditioning can still be achieved as long as you are working within the target heart rate training zone you've established. To help elevate your heart rate if it's not in your zone, place more emphasis on weight-bearing moves that lower your center of gravity. Deepening knee flexion (bending motions) that use the large leg and buttocks muscles (quadriceps and hamstrings, and gluteals) and gesture actions of the upper body are ways to accomplish this.. A step-touch, lunge, the grapevine, marching, and vigorous walking in place, are all examples of low-impact moves.

The following is a list of characteristics of low-impact aerobics:

▶ Heart rate is kept in the target heart rate training zone.

▶ Moves can be modified if THR is not maintained.

▶ Any tempo music can be utilized.

▶ For faster tempos, cover less space.

▶ For slower tempos, cover more space.

▶ Keep feet closer to the ground to decrease impact.

▶ Use moves traveling from side-to-side and forward-and-back, so large muscles of legs and trunk are continuously used.

▶ Use controlled, vigorous arm movements to compensate for the reduction in the activity of the leg and back muscles when the height of hops and jumps is reduced. "Research has shown that up to 25 percent more work can be performed with the arms and legs combined, compared to work performed by the legs alone."[32]

▶ Avoid using the arms above shoulder level for extended periods of time. "Doing so necessitates extended isometric contractions of the arm and shoulder muscles and probably causes greater after-exercise soreness. In addition, holding the arms over the head raises blood pressure, and anyone with high blood pressure or a history of angina pectoralis should be discouraged from doing these movements."[33]

▶ Turn toes/knees out with wide legs.

▶ Raise and lower the center of gravity.

▶ Lateral moves: keep legs turned out.

▶ Angle of knee flexion: 90 degrees.

▶ Strengthen both vastus medialis (front, inner thigh) and hamstrings.

▶ Use adductor muscles for correct mechanics.[34]

Low impact aerobics (LIA) is generally *not recommended* for:

▶ Anyone who complains of knee discomfort during prolonged knee flexion.

▶ Individuals who have severely flattened or *pronated* feet. (Knee flexion, and some side-to-side movements in which one foot crosses in front of the other, tend to produce a shifting of the kneecap toward the outer side of the knee joint and increases stress.)

▶ Well-conditioned, injury-free individuals who are unable to achieve their target heart rate, even in the most intense LIA programs. (Although many instructors use LIA exclusively in the interest of safety, conventional high-impact choreography may be acceptable for these participants — as long as they remain injury-free.)[35]

Combination High/Low-Impact Aerobics (CIA or Combo-Impact)

This impact style of choreography combines the characteristics for high- and low-impact movement and can be a safe and exciting blend of the two previously mentioned styles of impact. Combination high/low-impact choreography can be defined in two ways:[36]

1. *Routines that offer both a high-impact and low-impact version of a movement.* Programs that offer both work best in classes with mixed fitness levels, so that individual participants can select the amount of impact that is appropriate for them. A beginner in such a program, therefore, may choose to perform the low-impact version, while an experienced dance-exerciser may feel more challenged by the high-impact movements.

2. *Routines combining a series of varied high-impact and a series of varied low-impact movements.* This style lends itself well to classes of experienced aerobic dance-exercisers whose primary concern is to improve cardiorespiratory fitness, while minimizing the risk of injury.

Combo-impact aerobics presents you with a wide range of choices and possibilities. It allows you, personally, to individualize how much physical stress you choose to safely experience at various times and stages of your life according to your fitness level, personal goals, and special interests. Especially if you are a beginner, coming off an illness or injury, obese, older, or a pregnant woman, you'll want to choose the less biomechanically stressful low-impact movements.

Athletes in training and well-conditioned injury-free individuals may choose the high-impact movements and series more frequently, or even exclusively. As another option, they may wish to blend their HIA and LIA techniques into the *moderate-impact aerobic* (MIA) style explained later.

The unique feature of a combination approach is that you are familiar with all of the movement possibilities and can then choose the impact that best fits your current life-style needs. It is recognized here, however, that some people can never participate in the high-impact movements, due to permanent physical limitations.

A three-step process for interpreting high-impact steps into an acceptable low-impact movement (Figures 2.5–2.12) will be accomplished by:

① Lowering the foot impact.

② Increasing the arm movement.

③ Increasing the use of space.

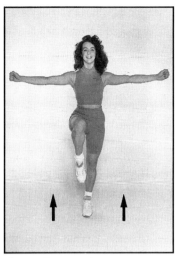
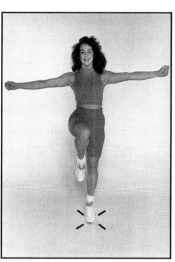
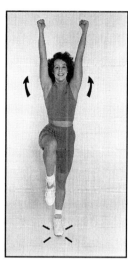
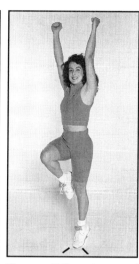

Figure 2.5. High-impact version of the step, knee-lift, hop; a vigorous move in which both feet leave the ground.

Figure 2.6. Impact is lowered by keeping the supporting foot flat on the floor.

Figure 2.7. Intensity is increased by raising the arms above the shoulders.

Figure 2.8. Increased use of space occurs when the knee is lifted higher (but no more than 90°) and exerciser lifts up onto the toe of the supporting leg.

① ② ③

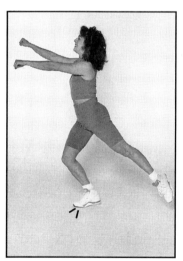
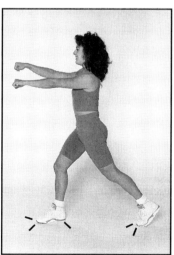
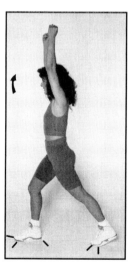
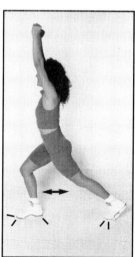

Figure 2.9. High-impact version of the lunge. The exerciser jumps high in the air when moving from side-to-side.

Figure 2.10. Impact is lowered by stepping outward instead of jumping.

Figure 2.11. Intensity is increased by raising the arms above the shoulders.

Figure 2.12. Increased use of space occurs by reaching out further, every step.

① ② ③

Step one of this process minimizes the impact, while steps two and three increase the intensity of the movement. The idea is to change one element at a time. First, lower the foot impact by keeping the feet closer to the floor. Second, exaggerate the original arm movement. Finally, increase the use of space by covering more ground with each step. Keen attention to the beat of the music becomes important when converting high-impact movement to low, to insure an injury-free workout.

Combining a series of varied high-impact and a series of varied low-impact movements will have fewer of the large upward impacts that are typical of a HIA program and will have fewer of the large side-to-side impacts that are typical of many LIA programs. A key to remember is that it is the sum total of all the stresses on the various vulnerable parts of the body that determines whether or not injury occurs.

Moderate-Impact Aerobics (MIA)

This is the fourth and the newest alternative style of impact-aerobics currently being used. It was designed as the result of laboratory and dance-exercise class research done at San Diego State University.[37] By adapting the gesture style (non-weight bearing body parts) and foot impact, this choreographic style combines the best elements of both HIA and LIA, for movements that keep the intensity needed to maintain target heart rate, while reducing foot-impact forces.

The key technique to master is called *plyometric*.[38] At least one foot remains in contact with the ground most of the time in order to reduce potentially injurious stresses on the body. However, the center of gravity of the body rises and falls almost as much as it does during HIA, thus avoiding prolonged knee flexion.[39] This raising and lowering of the center of gravity, by extending the hip, knee, and ankle joints without actually leaving the floor, requires *work*, the expenditure of energy. This will provide for relatively high exercise intensity.

Plyometric technique has been used for many years by athletes, in such sports as track and skiing, to increase power in a workout. These athletes have used plyometric techniques to increase their springing or bounding abilities. For example, picture yourself engaged in either sport and landing and recovering after a forceful jump move. When you lift and spring off the ground, that action is called plyometric. You are in fact forcefully loading the weight as you jump and then have a powerful unloading, or springing out of this move.[40]

Although this is a very effective method to increase power, it can be very stressful to the musculo-skeletal system of the average person. So in moderate-impact aerobics this plyometric principle of power in movement will be used, but you will load the weight with much less force by simply bending or flexing the knees and the hips, and then springing out of this position. This allows you to safely increase the intensity, and also safely increase power in your leg and hip muscles.

In many LIA routines, the emphasis is placed on flexing the knees so that the body is lowered and then raised to an erect position. This can be stressful to the knees of some participants. In addition, many beginners have found that this *down-up* movement is rather unnatural and requires a great deal of concentration. However, if the amount of knee flexion is decreased and *emphasis is placed on extending the knees and ankle joints without the feet actually leaving the floor* — as in moderate-impact aerobics — the center of gravity can be raised and lowered very effectively. The physiological cost of this is quite high, but the bouncy motions are comfortable and stimulating for many participants.[41]

Here's an example of *stepping-in-place*, clarifying the differences of the three distinct methods of impact:

▶ **High-impact aerobics:** Jogging — both feet off the ground for a brief moment.

▶ **Low-impact aerobics:** Marching — one foot always in contact with the floor.

▶ **Moderate-impact aerobics** using plyometric techniques that uses the lift and spring action (See Figure 2.13).

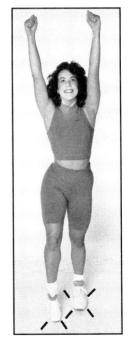

Figure 2.13. Keeping your right foot flat on the floor, raise your left foot until the tip of your left toe is just barely in contact with the ground. Now alternate the position of the feet to the same tempo that you used for the two previous movements. Lift your body as high as possible as you shift your weight from foot to foot by using the full range of motion of your ankle joints and moderate amounts of knee flexion and extension. Make certain that the heel of the supporting foot is pressed to the floor to maintain a good range of motion of the ankle joint.

The main difference between the high-impact jogging and moderate-impact version is the *rate at which the force is increased on the foot.* Even though the final load on the foot for the MIA step is close in magnitude to that for the HIA step, the load was increased much more gradually during the MIA step.

Researchers believe that when high levels of force are exerted on the feet very suddenly, the human body is vulnerable to injury. The body is equipped with reflex mechanisms that can control muscle contractions to protect it from mechanical stress. However, damage can occur if the forces reach high levels before the reflex mechanisms can provide protection. In practical terms, the springlike motions of MIA are less jarring than the high-impact versions because the body is raised and lowered with control. In HIA, the body is under less control as it falls freely, colliding suddenly with the floor.[42]

Guidelines For Using Moderate-Impact Aerobics

1. Begin movements by lifting your body upwards, rising onto the balls of your feet. Complete each step, whenever possible, by lowering your heels and gently pressing them against the floor. This pressing action produces the spring-like motion that is characteristic of MIA steps. It is the lifting and lowering of the center of gravity that increases exercise intensity.

2. Concentrate on leaving at least one foot on the floor most of the time. The purpose of MIA is to reduce the magnitude of impact. Steps such as MIA jogs, jumps, and twists are performed with both feet on the floor, either bearing the weight on both feet, as in a jump, or bearing it on one foot with the second foot lightly touching the floor, as in a twisting step.

    MIA steps that require lifting one foot off the floor, such as kicks and knee-lifts, must be carefully timed so that the airborne foot is back on the floor before the opposite foot leaves the ground.

3. Exercise intensity can be increased by directionally traveling across the floor and using the arms through a wide range of movement.

4. To adapt your present LIA or HIA moves to MIA, concentrate on taking the movement up and down while keeping one foot on the floor most of the time. (Keep in mind that not all LIA and HIA steps can be modified to suit MIA. Practice and common sense will help you determine which steps adjust best.) Examples of steps that adapt well to MIA include heel-jacks, jogs, jumps, kicks, knee-lifts, ponies, step-touches, and twists.

5. For variety, mix MIA with LIA and HIA steps.

6. Since the ankle joint is used through a wider range of motion with MIA than with HIA and LIA, it is particularly important to strengthen the tibialis anterior (shin area), and stretch the gastrocnemius and soleus (posterior, lower leg area) muscles during your warm-up and cool-down. These precautions will help prevent tightness of the calf and muscle imbalance.[43]

CALORIC EXPENDITURE OF AEROBICS

Recent research has indicated that, if all of the variables are carefully attended to and duplicated, aerobics can cause substantial energy expenditure of over 12 kcal/min, with no significant difference in caloric expenditure between low- and high-impact routines (if these routines are duplicated in style, content, and energy level).[44] This study was carried out using certified instructors (IDEA Foundation and/or AFAA) and involved two 11-minute sequences of high-impact and low-impact aerobic dance-exercise, at the tempo of 148 bpm. For those individuals concerned with weight management it is, therefore, exciting to conclude that one can engage in high- and/or low-impact moves and still significantly expend energy and burn calories!

Since the average peak force of LIA can result in impact forces of approximately 1½ times your weight and HIA can result in foot impact approximately 3 times your weight,[45] the impact that you choose can be important — especially if you have physical limitations (i.e., obese, pregnant, joint-injury prone). This choice of impact does not have to be made in regards to caloric expenditure, so be sure you understand all the pros and cons mentioned in this chapter before you choose your impact-style of expression.

TOTAL PHYSICAL FITNESS: A CHOICE!

It takes dedication to personal excellence to achieve physical fitness. There are few shortcuts, but many pleasurable alternatives. Once achieved, you must continue to make choices that maintain your fitness for a lifetime. Fitness is a journey — a continual process — not just one briefly achieved destination. You'll find that maintaining fitness is a lot easier, than initially achieving it. You will also discover that the less physically fit you are, the longer it will take you to become fit.

The total physical fitness journey requires

▶ seeking valid information;

▶ establishing your *starting points;*

▶ setting reasonable and challenging goals;

▶ monitoring your daily progress; and

▶ continually making self-disciplined choices from the imaged pictures you make in your head and your self-talk, to the motivated aerobic exercise moves you make.

You alone are the Captain of your ship.

You alone control the choices.

No one, and nothing else

can do it for you . . . .

Enjoy the journey!

Chapter 3

Establishing Your Program Starting Points: Fitness Testing

The next step in the journey toward achieving and then maintaining physical fitness for a lifetime involves establishing your current fitness *starting points* in the five component areas by using various scientific test and assessment procedures. Clearly knowing yourself in terms of your past history, risk factors, and present physical status will assist you in developing a lifetime fitness plan. It will enable you to not only realistically and safely set achievable short-term fitness goals, but will also serve to provide the basis for continually motivating you to adhere to the program you do establish, in order to achieve your long-range and lifetime fitness goals.

You may find initially that it can be very painful and devastating to realize that you are out of shape and test poorly on a laboratory or field stress test, are clinically labeled obese when you thought you were only a little bit overweight, mechanically have poor posture, or are below average in both your flexibility level and your muscular strength and endurance level for the various joints and muscle groups of your body. No one really wants to see or hear or feel scientific results that label them inferior or below the norm. But having the determination and courage to find out just where you are at the outset, and then with time and dedication, progressing to the point where your post-assessment test numbers represent an excellent state of fitness and well-being is very motivating and is the ink needed to permanently blueprint your desired changes for a lifetime! Enjoy getting started on your change process through the testing and assessment of your starting points in the five components of physical fitness.

YOUR PHYSICAL ACTIVITY READINESS

It's crucial to recognize that, in most instances, specific fitness testing is appropriate only after a medical history is taken. It is necessary to be screened for any potential problems that could occur during an assessment, as well as to determine if you should be considered for a specific exercise prescription.

The questions on Chart 9, "Your Physical Activity Readiness,"[1] do not provide an exhaustive medical history, but they do offer an essential basis for pretesting. If you answer "yes" to any of these questions, please inform your instructor immediately, and see a physician for clearance prior to performing a fitness assessment or engaging in an aerobics program. A thorough medical examination is the recommended way to make sure that your current state of health and your physical capacity are adequate to safely engage in fitness assessments or programs.

UNDERSTANDING FITNESS ASSESSMENTS

The purpose of an initial pre-course fitness assessment is to establish a baseline of information in each fitness component, with later evaluations compared with your initial results to determine the changes you've achieved. Realize the following assessment principles:

1. Nearly all assessment protocols result in estimated values for the fitness component being measured.

So consider the testing as merely an effective way to measure your improvement in your performance over time and not as an absolutely correct physiologic measurement or comparison.

2. By following consistent procedures of testing, i.e., using the same test, person administering it, instrument, time of day, etc., you are more assured of accuracy in measurement over time.

3. Record results and be sure you understand the values you get by asking questions.

ASSESSMENT #1: MEASURING AEROBIC CAPACITY

Pre-assessing your current status by having a thorough physical fitness exam will measure your heart's response to increasing amounts of exercise (work, stress) by measuring your ability to use oxygen.

Physical fitness can and should be measured in one of two ways at least every three years:

▶ A laboratory physical fitness test.

▶ A field test administered by you and a friend.

The Laboratory Physical Fitness Test

The "master key" to good health and exercising without fear is a properly conducted treadmill stress test to check out the precise condition of your heart.[2] There's a difference between physical fitness and health, and the treadmill stress ECG helps to make that distinction.[3]

Before you are given a treadmill stress test, a thorough screening will occur. This consists of: 1) obtaining a brief history and physical exam during which the technician listens to your heart and lungs; 2) a check for the use of drugs that are known to affect the ECG (i.e., various heart and hypertensive medications); 3) a check for a history of congenital or acquired heart disorders; and 4) an evaluation of the resting ECG (twelve-lead). Participating in this screening and background check will help to determine your risk factors. A risk factor is a feature in a person's heredity, background, or present lifestyle that increases the likelihood of developing coronary heart disease. Many risk factors are identified on Chart 9.

If no risk factors are present, an exercise test is not usually necessary below age thirty-five if guidelines mentioned in Chapter 2 are followed.

If symptoms of heart, lung, or metabolic disease are present, a maximum stress test is recommended for persons of any age, prior to the onset of a vigorous exercise program, and followed with tests every two years.[4]

Sub-Maximal vs Maximal Testing

Sub-maximal testing is accomplished by means of a physical fitness test (stress test) on a treadmill. Electrocardiogram leads transmit and record electrical (heart) impulses that are read on a machine and recorded on a strip of paper. You are tested only to approximately 150 beats per minute — not to exhaustion.

The ECG electrodes with leads are circular rubber discs that have wires attached to them. The discs are glued onto the chest and back at key locations so that various "pictures" of your heart, different angles and sides, can all be recorded at once. Usually between seven and ten electrodes are applied, depending on the laboratory's procedures or on the individual's specific needs.

You will probably be asked to walk at a pace of 3.3 miles per hour (90 meters per minute) on the treadmill. The grade will begin flat and will slowly increase in gradation, as if you were walking up a hill. Every minute the "hill" will become steeper and more difficult to climb. When your heart rate reaches 150 beats per minute, a record is made of the amount of time it took for you to arrive at that reading. Then, through an indirect method of extrapolation (projection of maximum results through having tested many others the same way in the past), your fitness ability is estimated.

Basically, the longer it takes your heart rate to reach 150 beats per minute, the more fit you are; the shorter it takes, the less fit you are. Sub-maximal fitness testing is usually used for persons who have no outstanding limitations known to them, and who are interested in starting an aerobics program.

Maximal testing procedures are administered if an individual's need is more specific (i.e., for diagnostic or research purposes). Maximum testing directly reveals how much oxygen you use, because you are tested to exhaustion. The "exhaustion" point is when you start to get markedly fatigued. Some researchers feel that maximum laboratory testing is the *only* really conclusive type to use.

Field Tests of Fitness

You may not have immediate access to a laboratory and qualified physiologists to monitor the results recorded with the treadmill method. Therefore, included here are field tests that have been developed to help you assess your own physical fitness by determining your current aerobic capacity.

This testing is easily conducted in an aerobics class setting.

The following information and Tables 3.1 and 3.2 were developed from Dr. Kenneth H. Cooper's book, *The Aerobics Program for Total Well-Being*.[5] Cooper's Twelve-Minute Test and 1.5-Mile Test are two that you can administer by yourself or with the help of a friend. Assess your cardiorespiratory endurance using one of these tests before you begin your aerobics program. Re-assess your cardiorespiratory efficiency eight weeks later. As aerobics becomes a lifetime activity for you, plan an ongoing assessment every two months. Compare your results with those from your first assessment. This will also help you set continual, life-long specific physical fitness goals.

Note

If you are over age thirty-five, it is strongly recommended that you start an aerobics program by first seeing your doctor, and then having a monitored laboratory-fitness test. Individuals with known cardiovascular, pulmonary, or metabolic disease should have a maximum stress test prior to beginning vigorous exercise at any age. These persons and persons with abnormal exercise tests should have a stress test annually.

Field Testing: Guidelines and Procedures

1 Before undertaking either of these tests, it is strongly recommended that previously physically inactive people participate in one to two weeks of walking and/or slow jogging before testing themselves.

2 Wear loose clothing in which you can freely sweat and a sport shoe that conforms to the guidelines suggested in Chapter 5.

3 Determine first which field test you plan to take. You can choose running with time or distance as the stopping point.

▶ If time is the stopping point, take the twelve-minute test.

▶ If distance is the stopping point, take the 1.5-mile test.

▶ If you feel rather strongly that you are really out of shape, the twelve-minute test will be easier because you run for only this amount of time. (It may take an individual twenty minutes to complete 1.5 miles.)

4 Be sure that you have a stopwatch or a second-hand on your watch, or that you are close to a wall timer.

5 Immediately before performing the test, spend five to ten minutes warming up the muscles (see Chapter 7).

6 Have a partner who is observing your testing, record your data on Chart 10 in the Appendix entitled, "Pre- & Post-Physical Fitness Testing and Appraisal Results," in the Pre-Test (A or B) section.

7 Run or walk (or combination) as quickly as you can for a total of twelve minutes or 1.5 miles. This is an all-out test of endurance.

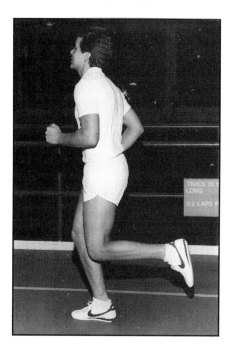

Figure 3.1.

8 When you stop, identify precisely the distance covered in miles and tenths of miles or time it took, and have your partner record it on Chart 10.

9 Be sure to cool down (see Chapter 7), by first walking slowly for several minutes, and then finish by performing cool-down stretching.

10 Interpret your results for the specific test that you used (Table 3-1 or 3-2).

11 Determine and circle your fitness level again on Chart 10.

12 At the conclusion of your course, re-assess your fitness on the same chart in the Post-Test (A or B) section and label your fitness level. What change did you experience from the Pre-Test to Post-Test?

TABLE 3.1   **Cooper's 12-Minute Walking/Running Test[6]**
Distance (Miles) Covered in 12 Minutes   **Use Appraisal A**

< Means less than; > means more than.

Fitness Category		13-19	20-29	30-39	40-49	50-59	60 +
				Age (years)			
I. Very Poor	(men)	<1.30	<1.22	<1.18	<1.14	<1.03	< .87
	(women)	<1.0	< .96	< .94	< .88	< .84	< .78
II. Poor	(men)	1.30-1.37	1.22-1.31	1.18-1.30	1.14-1.24	1.03-1.16	.87-1.02
	(women)	1.00-1.18	.96-1.11	.95-1.05	.88- .98	.84- .93	.78- .86
III. Fair	(men)	1.38-1.56	1.32-1.49	1.31-1.45	1.25-1.39	1.17-1.30	1.03-1.20
	(women)	1.19-1.29	1.12-1.22	1.06-1.18	.99-1.11	.94-1.05	.87- .98
IV. Good	(men)	1.57-1.72	1.50-1.64	1.46-1.56	1.40-1.53	1.31-1.44	1.21-1.32
	(women)	1.30-1.43	1.23-1.34	1.19-1.29	1.12-1.24	1.06-1.18	.99-1.09
V. Excellent	(men)	1.73-1.86	1.65-1.76	1.57-1.69	1.54-1.65	1.45-1.58	1.33-1.55
	(women)	1.44-1.51	1.35-1.45	1.30-1.39	1.25-1.34	1.19-1.30	1.10-1.18
VI. Superior	(men)	>1.87	>1.77	>1.70	>1.66	>1.59	>1.56
	(women)	>1.52	>1.46	>1.40	>1.35	>1.31	>1.19

TABLE 3.2   **Cooper's 1.5-Mile Run/Walk Test**
Time (Minutes)[7]   **Use Appraisal B**

< Means less than; > means more than.

Fitness Category		13-19	20-29	30-39	40-49	50-59	60 +
				Age (years)			
I. Very Poor	(men)	>15:31	>16:01	>16:31	>17:31	>19:01	>20:01
	(women)	>18:31	>19:01	>19:31	>20:01	>20:31	>21:01
II. Poor	(men)	12:11-15:30	14:01-16:00	14:44-16:30	15:36-17:30	17:01-19:00	19:01-20:00
	(women)	16:55-18:30	18:31-19:00	19:01-19:30	19:31-20:00	20:01-20:30	21:00-21:31
III. Fair	(men)	10:49-12:10	12:01-14:00	12:31-14:45	13:01-15:35	14:31-17:00	16:16-19:00
	(women)	14:31-16:54	15:55-18:30	16:31-19:00	17:31-19:30	19:01-20:00	19:31-20:30
IV. Good	(men)	9:41-10:48	10:46-12:00	11:01-12:30	11:31-13:00	12:31-14:30	14:00-16:15
	(women)	12:30-14:30	13:31-15:54	14:31-16:30	15:56-17:30	16:31-19:00	17:31-19:30
V. Excellent	(men)	8:37- 9:40	9:45-10:45	10:00-11:00	10:30-11:30	11:00-12:30	11:15-13:59
	(women)	11:50-12:29	12:30-13:30	13:00-14:30	13:45-15:55	14:30-16:30	16:30-17:30
VI. Superior	(men)	< 8:37	< 9:45	<10:00	<10:30	<11:00	<11:15
	(women)	<11:50	<12:30	<13:00	<13:45	<14:30	<16:30

13 Remember — for some beginners, the "good" performance level is very high. Do not be discouraged. You'll be pleased with your improvement as you participate in a regular aerobics program.

Fitness for Life

Attaining a level of physical fitness labeled "good" or "high" (lab tests), or "good", "excellent", or "superior" (field tests) does not mean that you have achieved a finished product or goal. Instead, you have found a method of getting in shape that must be continued for the rest of your life. If you discontinue your program completely, all your aerobic gains will be lost in ten weeks.[8]

The need for personal fitness must, therefore, result in a complete change in lifestyle. You must prioritize and program exercise into your busy weekly schedule for the rest of your life. A "yo-yo" concept of a ten-week class now, and maybe one a year later, just doesn't maintain fitness and a healthy heart!

ASSESSMENT #2: MUSCULAR ENDURANCE TESTING

Muscular strength and endurance represents the second of five total physical fitness components that are being tested for starting points. Although muscular strength and endurance are interrelated, a basic difference exists between the two. Strength is the capacity of a muscle to exert maximal force against a resistance. Endurance is the capacity of a muscle to exert submaximal force repeatedly over a period of time. Absolute strength is usually determined by the maximal amount of resistance (one repetition maximum or 1RM) that an individual can lift in a single effort. Because it requires access to a weight room and free weights or weight machines and some experience in weight training techniques, and is not as easily tested in an aerobics class, absolute strength will not be tested at this time.

Since muscular endurance, on the other hand, is commonly determined by the number of repetitions that an individual can perform against a submaximal resistance, or by the length of time that a given contraction can be sustained, it can easily and safely be tested in the aerobics class setting. The muscular endurance testing presented here consists of several different exercises that are used to determine the endurance of specific muscle groups. The advantage of this testing is that it requires just two pieces of equipment — a chinning bar and a sixteen-inch-high bench. Record your results from each exercise on Chart 11 in the Appendix entitled "Muscular Endurance Testing," under the score column.

Procedures for Muscular Endurance Testing[9]

1 Five different exercises are conducted during this testing and depending on the description of each one you will be asked to:

   ▶ perform a maximum number of continuous repetitions (Exercises II, IV, V);

   ▶ perform a maximum number of repetitions in the given period of time of one minute (Exercises I, VII);

   ▶ hold a particular contraction as long as possible (Exercises III, VI).

Perform each exercise as described and record results.

2 Refer now to your score results recorded on Chart 11. Consulting Table 3-3 Muscular Endurance Scoring look up your percentile ranking for each of your five exercises at the left margin. Record your percentile ranking now on Chart 11, Section A.

3 Total the percentile scores obtained for each exercise, and divide by five to obtain an average percentile rank score. Determine your overall muscular endurance fitness classification according to the average percentile rank scores on the bottom of Table 3-3. Record both your average score and classification on Chart 11, Section A.

4 Post-test yourself at the conclusion of the course and determine any change that has occurred in your overall muscular endurance fitness.

▌ Bent-Leg Sit-Up

Bend both legs at the knees at approximately ninety degrees. Having a partner hold your feet flat on the floor, attempt to do as many repetitions as possible in a one-minute period. At the start of each sit-up, the back of the head has to come in contact with the floor. At the top, at least one elbow must touch one knee (see Figures 3.2 and 3.3). One repetition is counted each time you complete the cycle and return back to the floor. Record repetitions.

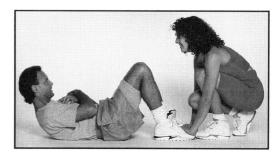

Figure 3.2. Step 1 - Lying down.

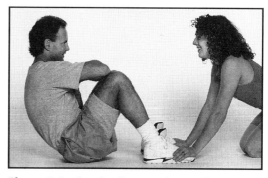

Figure 3.3. Step 2 - Sit up, with one elbow touching knee.

TABLE 3.3   **Muscular Endurance Scoring**

Test:	I Bent-Leg Sit-ups (1 Minute Maximum)		II Push-Ups (Reps)	III Static Push-Ups (In Seconds)		IV Pull-Ups (Reps)	V Modified Pull-Ups (Reps)	VI Flexed-Arm Hang (In Seconds)	VII Bench Jumps (Reps)	
Percentile Rank	Men	Women	Men	Men	Women	Men	Women	Women	Men	Women
95	50	36	53	97	38	14	43	34	38	28
90	47	33	49	72	35	12	40	28	36	26
80	44	30	44	67	32	10	36	19	34	24
70	41	28	41	63	30	9	33	14	33	22
60	39	26	38	60	28	8	30	10	31	21
50	37	24	35	57	26	7	28	8	30	20
40	35	22	32	54	24	6	26	6	29	19
30	33	20	29	51	22	5	23	4	27	18
20	30	18	26	47	20	4	20	2	26	16
10	27	15	21	42	17	2	16	1	24	14
5	24	12	17	37	14	0	13	0	22	12

Average Percentile Rank Score: **Muscular Endurance Fitness Classification:**

Average Percentile Rank Score		Classification
80 +	=	Excellent
60-79	=	Good
40-59	=	Average
20-39	=	Fair
< 19	=	Poor

Information reproduced with permission from Hockey, R. V. *Physical Fitness: The Pathway to Healthful Living.* St. Louis: Times Mirror/Mosby College Publishing, 1985

II Push-Up

The men perform as many continuous push-ups as possible. The body must be kept straight, the chest must touch the floor each time, and arms must be fully extended at the end of each repetition (see Figures 3.4 and 3.5). One rep is counted each time you complete cycle and return up to full arm extension. Record repetitions.

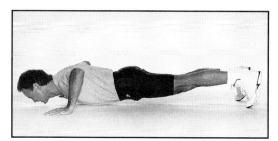

Figure 3.4. Step 1 - Chest touching floor.

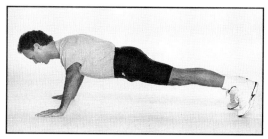

Figure 3.5 - Step 2 - Arms fully extended at end of rep.

III   Static Push-Up

Men and women alike perform a static push-up for as long as possible. This is done by lowering the body until the arms are flexed to ninety degrees or less (two or three inches above the floor) (see Figure 3.6). The entire body must be kept straight and off the floor with the exception of hands and feet. Use a timer and record the number of seconds the position is held.

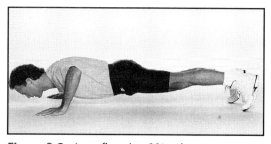

Figure 3.6. Arms flexed to 90° or less.

IV   Pull-Up

Men perform as many continuous pull-ups as possible. Grasp the bar with the palms forward. On each repetition, the chin has to raise above the bar (see Figure 3.7). The knees cannot be raised, nor are you allowed to kick with the legs when attempting the pull-ups. Record repetitions.

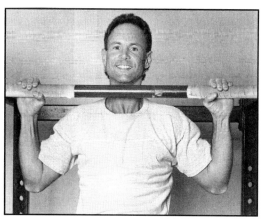

Figure 3.7. On each rep, chin raises above the bar.

V Modified Pull-Up

Women perform a modified pull-up by using a bar chest high, grasping the bar with palms forward, and sliding the feet under until the arms form a right angle with the body. Conduct as many continuous repetitions as possible, touching the bar with the chin or forehead on each repetition (Figure 3.8). Record repetitions.

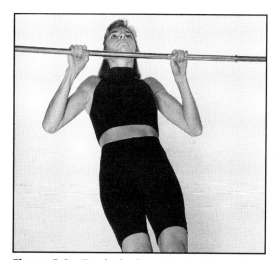

Figure 3.8. Touch the bar with the chin or forehead on each rep.

VI Flexed-Arm Hang

Women perform a flexed-arm hang by raising the chin to the level of the bar and holding this position as long as possible (Figure 3.9). Time stops once the chin cannot be kept level with the bar. Record the number of seconds the position is held.

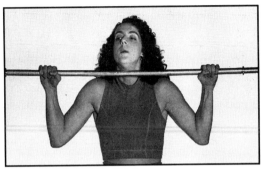

Figure 3.9. Raise chin to the bar and hold this position as long as possible.

VII Bench Jumps

Using a sixteen-inch bench, attempt to jump up onto and down from the bench as many times as possible in a one-minute period (Figure 3.10). If you cannot jump the full minute, you may step up and down. A repetition is counted each time both feet return to the floor. Record repetitions.

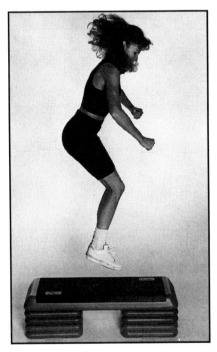

Figure 3.10. Jump up and down as many times as possible in one minute.

ASSESSMENT #3: FLEXIBILITY TESTING

Flexibility is the ability of a specific joint and its corresponding muscle groups to move freely through its full range of motion. It is reflected in each individual's ability to bend and stretch at various specific joints. Since total range of motion about a joint is highly specific and the range varies greatly from one joint to the other and also from one person to another, it is rather difficult to precisely indicate how much flexibility is ideal overall.

It is important, however, for the general population in an aerobics class to have some indication of how flexible their lower back and hamstring (posterior, upper leg area) muscles are, since this area is quite significantly used in all aerobic activities. One key exercise testing the flexibility of this area entitled The Modified Sit-and-Reach Test will be administered here.

Procedures for the Modified Sit-and-Reach Test

Note:

Some warm up stretching of this area is advised before this test is administered.

1 Place a yardstick on top of a bench-step approximately twelve inches high (i.e., like one Sports Step™ and four support blocks).

2 Remove your shoes and sit on the floor with your hips, back, and head against a wall and your legs fully extended, with the soles of your feet flat against the bench.

3 As shown in Figure 3.11, place your hands on top of each other, and reach forward as far as possible keeping your head and back against the wall.

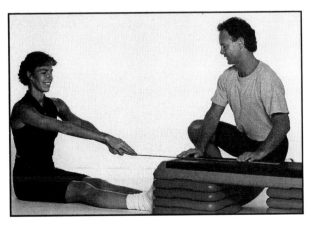

Figure 3.11. Determining the starting position.

4 Instructor or partner slides the yardstick along the top of the bench until the end touches your fingertips. The yardstick is now held firmly in place, until your results are recorded.

5 Allow your back and head to come off the wall. Slowly stretch forward as far as possible along the top of the yardstick. Hold the position (see Figure 3.12) for several seconds, as the instructor or partner determines the exact total number of inches you reached to the nearest one-half inch. Mentally note results.

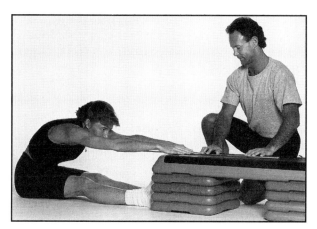

Figure 3.12. Modified Sit-and-Reach Test.

6 Repeat this procedure two more times and use the average of the three trials as your Modified Sit-and-Reach Test score. Using Table 3-4, and according to your age and gender, determine both your percentile rank and flexibility classification for this test.[10] Record your results on Chart 11, Section B.

Note:

Unlike the traditional Sit-and-Reach Test, the modified protocol used for this test varies in that the arm and leg lengths are taken into consideration to determine your score. In the original test procedures, the fifteen-inch mark of the yardstick is always set at the edge of the box where the feet are placed. This procedure does not differentiate between an individual with long arms and short legs and someone with short arms and long legs. All other factors being equal, the individual with the longer arms and shorter legs would receive a better rating because of the structural advantage.[11]

ASSESSMENT #4: BODY COMPOSITION

Your body is composed of two weights: lean weight and fat weight. These two weights are also called your lean body mass or fat-free mass, and your fat mass. Lean weight is composed primarily of your

TABLE 3.4   Percentile Ranks for the Modified Sit-and-Reach Test[10]

Men Percentile Rank	Age Category				Women Percentile Rank	Age Category				Flexibility Fitness Categories	
	<18	19-35	36-49	50>		<18	19-35	36-49	50>	Percentile Rank	Fitness Category
99	20.8	20.1	18.9	16.2	99	22.6	21.0	19.8	17.2	81>	Excellent
95	19.6	18.9	18.2	15.8	95	19.5	19.3	19.2	15.7		
90	18.2	17.2	16.1	15.0	90	18.7	17.9	17.4	15.0	61-80	Good
80	17.8	17.0	14.6	13.3	80	17.8	16.7	16.2	14.2		
70	16.0	15.8	13.9	12.3	70	16.5	16.2	15.2	13.6	41-60	Average
60	15.2	15.0	13.4	11.5	60	16.0	15.8	14.5	12.3		
50	14.5	14.4	12.6	10.2	50	15.2	14.8	13.5	11.1	21-40	Fair
40	14.0	13.5	11.6	9.7	40	14.5	14.5	12.8	10.1		
30	13.4	13.0	10.8	9.3	30	13.7	13.7	12.2	9.2	<20	Poor
20	11.8	11.6	9.9	8.8	20	12.6	12.6	11.0	8.3		
10	9.5	9.2	8.3	7.8	10	11.4	10.1	9.7	7.5		
05	8.4	7.9	7.0	7.2	05	9.4	8.1	8.5	3.7		
01	7.2	7.0	5.1	4.0	01	6.5	2.6	2.0	1.5		

▓▓ High physical fitness standard

▒▒ Health fitness standard

bones, muscles, and internal organs. Fat weight is just that. It is stored energy and protection that you are wearing for present and future use. The amount of each type of weight that you carry is important to know to understand what is best for the health of your heart and lungs (i.e., cardiorespiratory system).

Understanding Fat Weight and Lean Weight

Body fat can be classified into two types, essential fat and storage fat. The essential fat is needed for normal physiological functions, and without it, your health begins to deteriorate. This essential fat constitutes about 3 percent of the total fat in men and 10 to 12 percent in women. The percentage is higher in women because it includes gender-related fat, such as that found in the breast tissue, the uterus, and other gender-related areas of fat deposits.

Storage fat constitutes the fat that is stored in adipose tissue, mostly beneath the skin (subcutaneous fat) and around major organs in the body. This fat serves three basic functions: 1) as an insulator to retain body heat, 2) as energy substrate for metabolism, and 3) as padding against physical trauma to the body. The amount of storage fat does not differ between men and women except that men tend to store fat around the waist, and women more so around the hips and thighs.[12]

Your lean weight, on the other hand, is your fat-free weight or mass. It begins to weigh less after maturity when you stop growing at a certain steady pace every year. This is one of the unique aging processes. To slow down the aging processes and maintain your strength and lean weight, you'll need to incorporate a regular muscular strength and endurance program called strength or weight training as a part of your total fitness program. For each individual's amount of lean tissue, a certain percentage of fat can be "worn" to maintain ideal cardiorespiratory efficiency and minimize risk factors associated with heart disease. This is the key point to be made in regards to this fitness component, and the reason why it is assessed and improved or maintained by the exercise and eating programs you establish.

You may find that you are perhaps wearing less than a suggested ideal percentage of fat than is listed. This doesn't matter unless: 1) you are malnourishing yourself, or 2) you cosmetically wish to look heavier. A number of people don't wear the listed ideal percentages. Take for example endurance athletes like marathon runners or Olympic gymnasts, both of whom do not carry the suggested ideal percentages. They carry much less. They simply burn it off and don't carry the excess. They usually eat right

to provide the necessary nutrients and energy and thus display a firm, trim, toned look. The wobbly-fat gelatin look is absent from these extremely physical people, and yet they stay well.

In contrast are the anorexic individuals who exhibit the starvation disease, anorexia nervosa. They also may carry less than the suggested ideal percentage of body fat and accomplish this feat through a process of also eliminating their lean weight. They desire a trim look but go about it in a way that is against all physiological principles of proper weight loss. To them, weight loss means dropping pounds to be slim at all costs, no matter what kind of weight it is, fat or lean. This is an extremely deterimental way to lose weight. To enable individuals to understand healthy slimness and unhealthy slimness, an indepth look at weight management is presented in Chapter 10.

Determining Your Body Composition

You cannot determine the amount of body fat and lean weight that a person has by merely looking at them (see Figure 3-13). An assessment of body

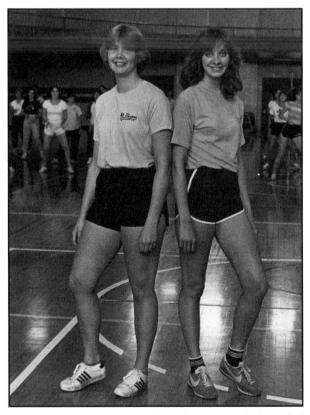

Figure 3.13. It is impossible to determine "ideal weight" just by looking at someone. Both of these college women are approximately 5'10" tall and are carrying the same percentage of body fat (28%) on their individual leans. At left, Paula's ideal weight is 145. On the right, Jill's ideal weight is 114.

composition involves determining as precisely as possible an individual's body fat and lean body weight. Such an assessment allows an accurate estimate to be made of what an individual's ideal weight should be. This is important, since the traditional approach of using standardized weight tables adjusted for gender, height, and frame size has been shown to be grossly inaccurate for a rather large percentage of the population. The ideal weight within any one category of these tables can vary up to twenty-two pounds. It is not unusual for an individual to fall within the normal range for his or her category but to actually have ten to thirty pounds of excess body fat.

Currently, measurement techniques have been sought to more accurately determine whether an individual is overweight (overfat) or obese and then quantify exactly by how much. A variety of techniques are available:

▶ Measuring skinfold thickness

▶ Analysis by electrical impedence

▶ Underwater weighing (specific gravity)

▶ Using both skinfold thickness and anthropometric measures of bone thickness or girth measurements or both

▶ Near-infrared interactance

Because of ease of use in an aerobics class setting and availability of equipment, only the first technique will be fully detailed here. This fitness component called body composition will be assessed now, and will determine your lean weight mass, the percentage of body fat that you're carrying, and then establish an estimated ideal body weight that is best for your cardiorespiratory health.

Measuring Skinfold Thickness

The assessment of body composition using skinfold thickness is based on the principle that approximately 50 percent of the fatty tissue in the body is deposited directly beneath the skin. If this tissue is estimated validly and reliably, a good indication of percent body fat can be obtained.

This test is performed with the aid of a precision instrument called a skinfold caliper. Three specific sites must be measured with the calipers and then added together to reflect the total percentage of fat you currently have. Small variations in measurements on the same subject may occur when these are taken by different professionals. Therefore, it is recommended that pre- and post-measurements be conducted by the same technician.

The procedures for assessing percent body fat using the 3-Site Skinfold Testing follows:

1 Select the proper anatomical sites. For men, test the chest, abdomen, and thigh (Figure 3.14). For women, the triceps, suprailium, and thigh areas are tested (Figures 3.15 and 3.16). All measurements should be taken on the right side of the body with the subject standing. The correct anatomical landmarks for skinfolds are:

Men

Chest:	A diagonal fold halfway between the shoulder crease and the nipple.
Abdomen:	A vertical fold taken about one inch to the right of the umbilicus.
Thigh:	A vertical fold on the front of the thigh, midway between the knee and hip.

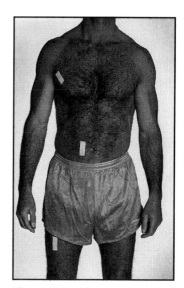

Figure 3.14. Proper anatomical sites for men.

Women

Triceps:	A vertical fold on the back of the upper arm, halfway between the shoulder and the elbow.
Suprailium:	A diagonal fold above the crest of the ilium (on the side of the hip)
Thigh:	A vertical fold on the front of the thigh, midway between the knee and hip.

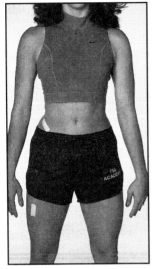
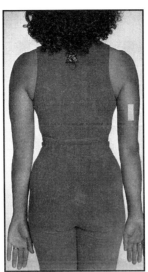

Figure 3.15.   **Figure 3.16.**
Proper anatomical sites for women.

2 The technician will measure you by grasping a thickness of your skin in the key locations just mentioned, with a thumb and forefinger, and pulling the fold slightly away from the muscular tissue. The calipers are held perpendicular to the fold, and the measurement is taken one-half inch below the finger hold. Each site is measured three times and the values are read to the nearest .1 to .5 mm. The average of the two closest readings is recorded as your final value. The readings will be taken without delay to avoid excessive compression of the skinfold. Releasing and re-grabbing the skinfold is required between readings.

3 When doing pre- and post-assessments, the measurement should be conducted at the same time of day. The best time is early in the morning to avoid hydration changes resulting from activity or exercise.

4 Your percent fat is obtained by adding together all three skinfold measurements and looking up the respective values on Tables 3-5 for women, 3-6 for men under forty, and 3-7 for men over forty. Record the numbers from each skinfold grab and your percent fat on Chart 12 in the Appendix entitled "Body Composition Assessment", Section A.

Lean Weight and Recommended/Ideal Weight Determined

After finding out your percent body fat, you can determine your current body composition classification according to Table 3 8.[16] In this table you will find the health fitness and the high physical fitness percent fat standards. For example, the recommended health fitness fat percentage for a twenty-year-old female is 28 percent or less. The health fitness standard is established at the point where there seems to be no detriment to health in terms of percent body fat. A high physical fitness range for this same woman would be between 18 and 23 percent. The high physical fitness standard does not mean that you cannot be somewhat below this number. As mentioned earlier, many highly trained athletes measurements are below the percentages set. However, the 3 percent essential fat for men and 12 percent for women are the lower limits for people to maintain good health. Below these percentages, normal physiologic functions can be seriously impaired.

In addition, some experts point out that a little storage fat (over the essential fat) is better than none at all. As a result, the health and high fitness standards for percent fat in Table 3.8 are set higher than the minimum essential fat requirements, at a point that is conducive to optimal health and well-being. Additionally, because lean tissue decreases with age, one extra percentage point is allowed for every additional decade of life.

Note: Your recommended body weight is computed based on the selected health or high fitness fat percentage for your respective age and gender. Your decision to select a desired fat percentage should be based on your current percent body fat and your personal health-fitness goals and objectives. To compute your own recommended or ideal body weight, see Chart 12, Section B, in the Appendix entitled, "Determining Recommended/Ideal Body Weight." Remember to refer back to Table 3-8 when selecting a desired body fat percentage (Step 3).

ASSESSMENT 5: POSTURE EVALUATION

Correct body positioning underlies all the exercise activities and movements that you'll ever do. The primary concern is for the safety of your spine and the various joints of the body. When movements are performed correctly so undue (negative) stress is not placed on the body, you'll experience enjoyment with your exercise program and be relatively pain-free by choosing to move in a mechanically correct way.

TABLE 3.5 **Percent Fat Estimates for Women Calculated from Triceps, Suprailium, and Thigh Skinfold Thickness**

Sum of 3 Skinfolds	Age to the Last Year								
	Under 22	23 to 27	28 to 32	33 to 37	38 to 42	43 to 47	48 to 52	53 to 57	Over 58
23-25	9.7	9.9	10.2	10.4	10.7	10.9	11.2	11.4	11.7
26-28	11.0	11.2	11.5	11.7	12.0	12.3	12.5	12.7	13.0
29-31	12.3	12.5	12.8	13.0	13.3	13.5	13.8	14.0	14.3
32-34	13.6	13.8	14.0	14.3	14.5	14.8	15.0	15.3	15.5
35-37	14.8	15.0	15.3	15.5	15.8	16.0	16.3	16.5	16.8
38-40	16.0	16.3	16.5	16.7	17.0	17.2	17.5	17.7	18.0
41-43	17.2	17.4	17.7	17.9	18.2	18.4	18.7	18.9	19.2
44-46	18.3	18.6	18.8	19.1	19.3	19.6	19.8	20.1	20.3
47-49	19.5	19.7	20.0	20.2	20.5	20.7	21.0	21.2	21.5
50-52	20.6	20.8	21.1	21.3	21.6	21.8	22.1	22.3	22.6
53-55	21.7	21.9	22.1	22.4	22.6	22.9	23.1	23.4	23.6
56-58	22.7	23.0	23.2	23.4	23.7	23.9	24.2	24.4	24.7
59-61	23.7	24.0	24.2	24.5	24.7	25.0	25.2	25.5	25.7
62-64	24.7	25.0	25.2	25.5	25.7	26.0	26.2	26.4	26.7
65-67	25.7	25.9	26.2	26.4	26.7	26.9	27.2	27.4	27.7
68-70	26.6	26.9	27.1	27.4	27.6	27.9	28.1	28.4	28.6
71-73	27.5	27.8	28.0	28.3	28.5	28.8	29.0	29.3	29.5
74-76	28.4	28.7	28.9	29.2	29.4	29.7	29.9	30.2	30.4
77-79	29.3	29.5	29.8	30.0	30.3	30.5	30.8	31.0	31.3
80-82	30.1	30.4	30.6	30.9	31.1	31.4	31.6	31.9	32.1
83-85	30.9	31.2	31.4	31.7	31.9	32.2	32.4	32.7	32.9
86-88	31.7	32.0	32.2	32.5	32.7	32.9	33.2	33.4	33.7
89-91	32.5	32.7	33.0	33.2	33.5	33.7	33.9	34.2	34.4
92-94	33.2	33.4	33.7	33.9	34.2	34.4	34.7	34.9	35.2
95-97	33.9	34.1	34.4	34.6	34.9	35.1	35.4	35.6	35.9
98-100	34.6	34.8	35.1	35.3	35.5	35.8	36.0	36.3	36.5
101-103	35.2	35.4	35.7	35.9	36.2	36.4	36.7	36.9	37.2
104-106	35.8	36.1	36.3	36.6	36.8	37.1	37.3	37.5	37.8
107-109	36.4	36.7	36.9	37.1	37.4	37.6	37.9	38.1	38.4
110-112	37.0	37.2	37.5	37.7	38.0	38.2	38.5	38.7	38.9
113-115	37.5	37.8	38.0	38.2	38.5	38.7	39.0	39.2	39.5
116-118	38.0	38.3	38.5	38.8	39.0	39.3	39.5	39.7	40.0
119-121	38.5	38.7	39.0	39.2	39.5	39.7	40.0	40.2	40.5
122-124	39.0	39.2	39.4	39.7	39.9	40.2	40.4	40.7	40.9
125-127	39.4	39.6	39.9	40.1	40.4	40.6	40.9	41.1	41.4
128-130	39.8	40.0	40.3	40.5	40.8	41.0	41.3	41.5	41.8

Body density calculated based on the generalized equation for predicting body density of women developed by A. S. Jackson, M. L. Pollock, and A. Ward. *Medicine and Science in Sports and Exercise* 12:175-182, 1980. Percent body fat determined from the calculated body density using the Siri formula.[13]

TABLE 3.6 **Percent Fat Estimates for Men Under 40 Calculated from Chest, Abdomen, and Thigh Skinfold Thickness**

Sum of 3 Skinfolds	Under 19	20 to 22	23 to 25	26 to 28	29 to 31	32 to 34	35 to 37	38 to 40
				Age to the Last Year				
8-10	.9	1.3	1.6	2.0	2.3	2.7	3.0	3.3
11-13	1.9	2.3	2.6	3.0	3.3	3.7	4.0	4.3
14-16	2.9	3.3	3.6	3.9	4.3	4.6	5.0	5.3
17-19	3.9	4.2	4.6	4.9	5.3	5.6	6.0	6.3
20-22	4.8	5.2	5.5	5.9	6.2	6.6	6.9	7.3
23-25	5.8	6.2	6.5	6.8	7.2	7.5	7.9	8.2
26-28	6.8	7.1	7.5	7.8	8.1	8.5	8.8	9.2
29-31	7.7	8.0	8.4	8.7	9.1	9.4	9.8	10.1
32-34	8.6	9.0	9.3	9.7	10.0	10.4	10.7	11.1
35-37	9.5	9.9	10.2	10.6	10.9	11.3	11.6	12.0
38-40	10.5	10.8	11.2	11.5	11.8	12.2	12.5	12.9
41-43	11.4	11.7	12.1	12.4	12.7	13.1	13.4	13.8
44-46	12.2	12.6	12.9	13.3	13.6	14.0	14.3	14.7
47-49	13.1	13.5	13.8	14.2	14.5	14.9	15.2	15.5
50-52	14.0	14.3	14.7	15.0	15.4	15.7	16.1	16.4
53-55	14.8	15.2	15.5	15.9	16.2	16.6	16.9	17.3
56-58	15.7	16.0	16.4	16.7	17.1	17.4	17.8	18.1
59-61	16.5	16.9	17.2	17.6	17.9	18.3	18.6	19.0
62-64	17.4	17.7	18.1	18.4	18.8	19.1	19.4	19.8
65-67	18.2	18.5	18.9	19.2	19.6	19.9	20.3	20.6
68-70	19.0	19.3	19.7	20.0	20.4	20.7	21.1	21.4
71-73	19.8	20.1	20.5	20.8	21.2	21.5	21.9	22.2
74-76	20.6	20.9	21.3	21.6	22.0	22.2	22.7	23.0
77-79	21.4	21.7	22.1	22.4	22.8	23.1	23.4	23.8
80-82	22.1	22.5	22.8	23.2	23.5	23.9	24.2	24.6
83-85	22.9	23.2	23.6	23.9	24.3	24.6	25.0	25.3
86-88	23.6	24.0	24.3	24.7	25.0	25.4	25.7	26.1
89-91	24.4	24.7	25.1	25.4	25.8	26.1	26.5	26.8
92-94	25.1	25.5	25.8	26.2	26.5	26.9	27.2	27.5
95-97	25.8	26.2	26.5	26.9	27.2	27.6	27.9	28.3
98-100	26.6	26.9	27.3	27.6	27.9	28.3	28.6	29.0
101-103	27.3	27.6	28.0	28.3	28.6	29.0	29.3	29.7
104-106	27.9	28.3	28.6	29.0	29.3	29.7	30.0	30.4
107-109	28.6	29.0	29.3	29.7	30.0	30.4	30.7	31.1
110-112	29.3	29.6	30.0	30.3	30.7	31.0	31.4	31.7
113-115	30.0	30.3	30.7	31.0	31.3	31.7	32.0	32.4
116-118	30.6	31.0	31.3	31.6	32.0	32.3	32.7	33.0
119-121	31.3	31.6	32.0	32.3	32.6	33.0	33.3	33.7
122-124	31.9	32.2	32.6	32.9	33.3	33.6	34.0	34.3
125-127	32.5	32.9	33.2	33.5	33.9	34.2	34.6	34.9
128-130	33.1	33.5	33.8	34.2	34.5	34.9	35.2	35.5

Body density calculated based on the generalized equation for predicting body density of men developed by A. S. Jackson, M. L. Pollock. *British Journal of Nutrition* 40:497-504, 1978. Percent body fat determined from the calculated body density using the Siri formula.[14]

TABLE 3.7 **Percent Fat Estimates for Men Over 40 Calculated from Chest, Abdomen, and Thigh Skinfold Thickness**

Sum of 3 Skinfolds	Age to the Last Year							
	41 to 43	44 to 46	47 to 49	50 to 52	53 to 55	56 to 58	59 to 61	Over 62
8-10	3.7	4.0	4.4	4.7	5.1	5.4	5.8	6.1
11-13	4.7	5.0	5.4	5.7	6.1	6.4	6.8	7.1
14-16	5.7	6.0	6.4	6.7	7.1	7.4	7.8	8.1
17-19	6.7	7.0	7.4	7.7	8.1	8.4	8.7	9.1
20-22	7.6	8.0	8.3	8.7	9.0	9.4	9.7	10.1
23-25	8.6	8.9	9.3	9.6	10.0	10.3	10.7	11.0
26-28	9.5	9.9	10.2	10.6	10.9	11.3	11.6	12.0
29-31	10.5	10.8	11.2	11.5	11.9	12.2	12.6	12.9
32-34	11.4	11.8	12.1	12.4	12.8	13.1	13.5	13.8
35-37	12.3	12.7	13.0	13.4	13.7	14.1	14.4	14.8
38-40	13.2	13.6	13.9	14.3	14.6	15.0	15.3	15.7
41-43	14.1	14.5	14.8	15.2	15.5	15.9	16.2	16.6
44-46	15.0	15.4	15.7	16.1	16.4	16.8	17.1	17.5
47-49	15.9	16.2	16.6	16.9	17.3	17.6	18.0	18.3
50-52	16.8	17.1	17.5	17.8	18.2	18.5	18.8	19.2
53-55	17.6	18.0	18.3	18.7	19.0	19.4	19.7	20.1
56-58	18.5	18.8	19.2	19.5	19.9	20.2	20.6	20.9
59-61	19.3	19.7	20.0	20.4	20.7	21.0	21.4	21.7
62-64	20.1	20.5	20.8	21.2	21.5	21.9	22.2	22.6
65-67	21.0	21.3	21.7	22.0	22.4	22.7	23.0	23.4
68-70	21.8	22.1	22.5	22.8	23.2	23.5	23.9	24.2
71-73	22.6	22.9	23.3	23.6	24.0	24.3	24.7	25.0
74-76	23.4	23.7	24.1	24.4	24.8	25.1	25.4	25.8
77-79	24.1	24.5	24.8	25.2	25.5	25.9	26.2	26.6
80-82	24.9	25.3	25.6	26.0	26.3	26.6	27.0	27.3
83-85	25.7	26.0	26.4	26.7	27.1	27.4	27.8	28.1
86-88	26.4	26.8	27.1	27.5	27.8	28.2	28.5	28.9
89-91	27.2	27.5	27.9	28.2	28.6	28.9	29.2	29.6
92-94	27.9	28.2	28.6	28.9	29.3	29.6	30.0	30.3
95-97	28.6	29.0	29.3	29.7	30.0	30.4	30.7	31.1
98-100	29.3	29.7	30.0	30.4	30.7	31.1	31.4	31.8
101-103	30.0	30.4	30.7	31.1	31.4	31.8	32.1	32.5
104-106	30.7	31.1	31.4	31.8	32.1	32.5	32.8	33.2
107-109	31.4	31.8	32.1	32.4	32.8	33.1	33.5	33.8
110-112	32.1	32.4	32.8	33.1	33.5	33.8	34.2	34.5
113-115	32.7	33.1	33.4	33.8	34.1	34.5	34.8	35.2
116-118	33.4	33.7	34.1	34.4	34.8	35.1	35.5	35.8
119-121	34.0	34.4	34.7	35.1	35.4	35.8	36.1	36.5
122-124	34.7	35.0	35.4	35.7	36.1	36.4	36.7	37.1
125-127	35.3	35.6	36.0	36.3	36.7	37.0	37.4	37.7
128-130	35.9	36.2	36.6	36.9	37.3	37.6	38.0	38.5

Body density calculated based on the generalized equation for predicting body density of men developed by A. S. Jackson, M. L. Pollock. *British Journal of Nutrition* 40:497-504, 1978. Percent body fat determined from the calculated body density using the Siri formula.[15]

TABLE 3.8   Body Composition Classification According to percent Body Fat[16]

MEN

Age	Excellent	Good	Moderate	Overweight	Obese
<19	12	12.5-17.0	17.5-22.0	22.5-27.0	27.5+
20-29	13	13.5-18.0	18.5-23.0	23.5-28.0	28.5+
30-39	14	14.5-19.0	19.5-24.0	24.5-29.0	29.5+
40-49	15	15.5-20.0	20.5-25.0	25.5-30.0	30.5+
50+	16	16.5-21.5	21.5-26.0	26.5-31.0	31.5+

WOMEN

Age	Excellent	Good	Moderate	Overweight	Obese
<19	17	17.5-22.0	22.5-27.0	27.5-32.0	32.5+
20-29	18	18.5-23.0	23.5-28.0	28.5-33.0	33.5+
30-39	19	19.5-24.0	24.5-29.0	29.5-34.0	34.5+
40-49	20	20.5-25.0	25.5-30.0	30.5-35.0	35.5+
50+	21	21.5-26.5	26.5-31.0	31.5-36.0	36.5+

■ High physical fitness standard
▒ Health fitness standard

By assessing your static (standing still) posture from both a side-view and a back-view, you'll begin to understand proper dynamic (moving through space) postures you'll be assuming with the various aerobic exercises you do. This will lead to both a safe and fun workout session.

Posture Evaluation Procedures

Picture time. Wear a swimsuit, runner's shorts, leotard and tights, or whatever is tight fitting, so that all of the body lines show. Take off your shoes, and if you have shoulder length hair either bring it forward off the shoulders, or tie it in the center back.

Have a photographer come and take two proof-size photos of you: 1) standing and facing sideward (Figure 3.17); and 2) from the back (Figure 3.18). In both views, have your arms at your sides and stand with your weight evenly distributed on both feet. Attach the photographs to Chart 13 in the Appendix, entitled, "Posture Problems: Detecting and Correcting." You will be able to use these for detecting and correcting any posture problems you might have. It usually takes the trained eye to make the most accurate assessment, so your instructor will probably want to fill out Chart 13 for the pre-assessment of

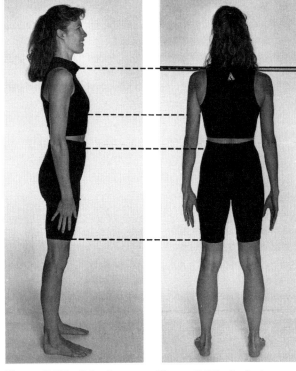

Figure 3.17. Side-view.   **Figure 3.18.** Back-view.

your posture. However, if you are asked to evaluate your own posture, wait to do this particular assessment until after you've read and understood Chapter 6. Follow these procedures:

1 Evaluate posture by first analyzing your side- and back-view photos.

2 Draw four horizontal lines connecting both inside photo edges to depict body segments and label these divisions:

▶ head/neck

▶ shoulder/upper back/chest

▶ lower back/abdomen

▶ pelvis – hips/thighs

▶ knees/ankles/feet.

3 Compare the criteria for balanced postures and those for the more common postural problems (as shown in Chapter 6, Figures 6.4 and 6.5) with your photos or by looking at yourself in a three-way mirror.

4 For item 1, to check if your body line is perpendicular through the center of your weight (i.e., the center of gravity), determine if a line goes from the tip of your ear through the center of your shoulder joint, slightly behind the center of your hip joint, behind your kneecap, and in front of your ankle joint. Do this by placing a straight-edge on your side-view photo and drawing a vertical line from one point of reference to the next. If the majority of your body falls in front of the line, then your body line will be backward (i.e., from a balanced, perpendicular line perspective); if the majority of your body falls behind the line, then your body line will be forward. You will also be able to tell immediately if your body line is straight (i.e., perpendicular to the ground) or a combination of zigzags.

5 Mark all of your pre-assessment checks on Chart 13.

6 When entire evaluation is completed, place an asterisk on your body segments that are unbalanced and need correction.

7 When you have completed your evaluation, have your instructor review your impressions and make her or his own additions and corrections.

8 At the conclusion of the course, evaluate your change and progress toward achieving good posture. This can best be achieved by again being photographed in your new standing posture, from both side- and back-views. Attach these new photos also to Chart 13, and mark post-assessment checks on the same chart, this time circling any postural corrections (i.e., the asterisks you have made since your pre-assessment). Any postural problems still remaining would be marked with an asterisk and doubled checked (✔✔). Your instructor may want to go over your final evaluation and give you suggestions for continual improvement.

SUMMARY

You have just completed assessing your initial starting points in the five physical fitness component areas. You know: 1) how fit your heart and lungs are (i.e., your aerobic capacity); 2) your muscular endurance fitness for key areas of the body; 3) the flexibility of your lower spine area; 4) your body composition in terms of lean weight and fat percentage, with an estimate of your recommended ideal weight established; and 5) how balanced your posture is.

With this information, it is now possible for you to establish goals in each of these component areas. Setting goals helps to keep you focused on daily improvement and positive change. It encourages a consistency in your fitness program and helps to keep you on target because without goals, there's nothing to shoot for!

Establish at least five short-term goals, one for each fitness component area you've assessed. Write each goal established on the individual assessment charts. Set each goal to be achieved by the end of this course, and remember to truly stretch yourself and your potential, in regards to what you are actually capable of achieving.

Chapter 4

Principles of Aerobics Programs

The foundation for understanding physical fitness has been set. Your mind is set, the basic new terminologies have been defined, and you have established your starting points in order to set your goals. It's now time to build upon this foundation that represents a safe, beneficial, and fun total fitness workout session.

AEROBICS PROGRAMMING

Each aerobics class workout session is structured into these basic segments:

1) a warm-up

2) aerobics

3) strength training

4) cool down, flexibility training, and relaxation.

Each of these basic segments are further structured into the following activities. Principles and guidelines are given for each. [1, 2, 3, 4, 5]

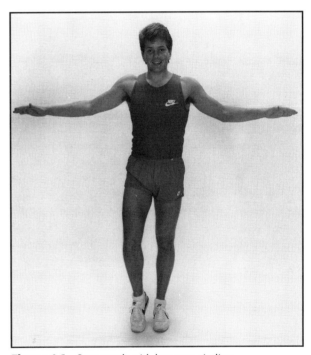

Figure 4.1. Step-touch with low arm circling.

I. Warm-Up Segment

The warm-up begins with activities that are active, low-level, rhythmic, limbering, standing, range-of-motion type of exercises that raise the body's core temperature slightly, initiate muscular movements and prepare you for more strenuous moves to come. Example: Step-touch with low arm-circling (Figure 4.1), or other gentle sweeping motions of low-intensity are good to initiate the warm-up. The time frame can be approximately 5 minutes.

Following the initial warm-up exercises, slow, sustained, static stretching is performed since the muscles, tendons, ligaments, and joints are loose and pliable. Static stretching is performed from head to toe (Figures 4.2 – 4.4). It is probably the most popular, easiest, and safest form of stretching available. It involves gradually stretching a muscle or muscle group to the point of limitation, then holding that position for approximately 15 seconds. The stretch is

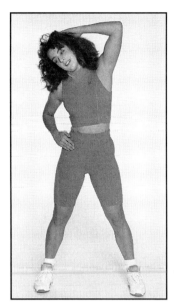

Figure 4.2.
Head drop to the side and press

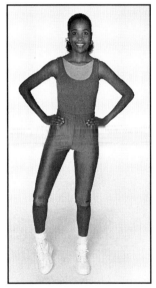 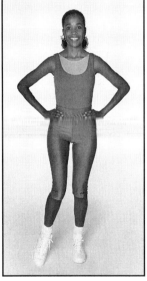

Figure 4.3.   Ankle Stretching.   **Figure 4.4.**

then repeated to the opposite side. Several repetitions of each stretch are performed. Static stretching is recommended when muscles are warm, which is after the initial active phase of the warm-up and later after intense physical activity.

Breathing Technique

Breathe continuously. Your entire system, especially your working muscles, constantly need oxygen. Holding your breath and turning red is never an appropriate way to exercise. While performing the warm-up and cool-down stretching (or any strengthening exercise), exhale when you stretch, by puckering your lips and breathing out, and inhale when you can relax your muscles.

Cue yourself: "breathe out and stretch"; "breathe in and relax."

The time frame for the warm-up stretching segment can be approximately 5 minutes.

II. Aerobics Segment

The aerobics segment can be sub-divided into six sections, each one focusing on the impact that you perform in relation to the heart rate intensity you are building, sustaining, or lowering and according to which phase of the hour you're in. At least two heart-rate checks should be monitored during the segment.

Low-Impact Aerobics Warm-up

These are simple, low-intensity moves that gradually increase your heart-rate. They start with the legs down low and arms below heart level. To gradually increase the intensity, first increase the range-of-motion of each movement, and then increase the use of air and floor space. For example: Step-touch in place with hand claps, punching, or (**Figure 4.5**) arms shoulder high with hands pointing in, and then both hands and toe-touch extending far out, to the side. Progress to a grapevine, using large arm reaches (Figures 4.6–4.9). The time frame can be approximately 5 minutes.

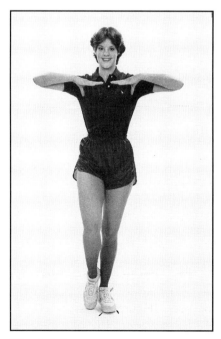

Figure 4.5.

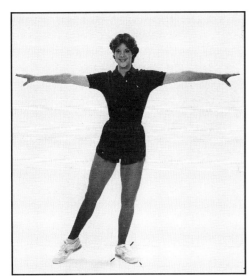

Figure 4.6.

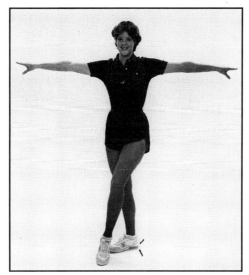

Figure 4.7.

The Grapevine

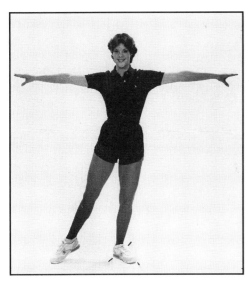

Figure 4.8.

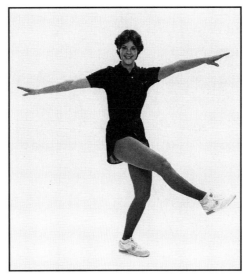

Figure 4.9.

Power Low-Impact Aerobics

These moves increase the load on the large muscles of the legs by bending and extending more, with the accent on the lifting or raising of the center of gravity while keeping at least one foot firmly on the floor and recovering with an ankle-flexion springing movement. Traveling through space is characteristic with these movements that really challenge the leg muscles. Examples are: strong low-impact bouncing and reaching with plyometrics (Figure 4.10), squats or plies (Figures 4.11 and 4.12), lunges (Figure 4.13), and power walking (Figure 4.14). The time frame can be approximately 10 minutes.)

High/Low-Impact Aerobics

Here you'll intersperse high-impact moves, where both feet may momentarily leave the floor, with low-impact moves, where one foot always remains on the floor. You'll raise your arms overhead more frequently, and raise the knees and feet up higher. A key point in this segment is that the intensity of the moves you choose must remain high so the heart-rate maintains the high but safe, training zone you've established for cardiorespiratory improvement. Not more than four high-impact repetitions are performed on the same leg at one time. The music speed will range between up to 160 BPM for

— Power Low-Impact —

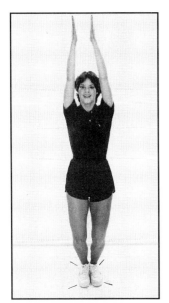

Figure 4.10.
Bouncing and reaching.

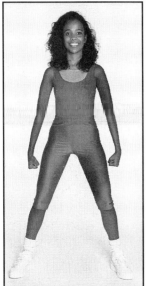

Figure 4.11. (Step 1).

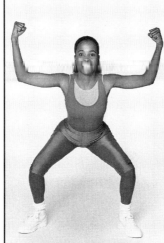

Figure 4.12. (Step 2) Squats.

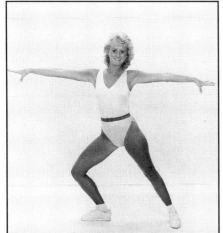

Figure 4.13.
Lunges.

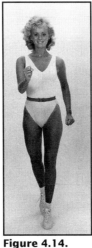

Figure 4.14.
Walk.

low-impact moves and up to 180 BPM for high-impact exercises. Examples are: two high impact jacks in the wide-stride-and-together leg and arm positions (Figures 4.15 and 4.16), followed by four, power low-impact pace-walking moves with forceful arms (Figure 4.17). The time frame can be approximately 15 minutes.

— High/Low-Impact —

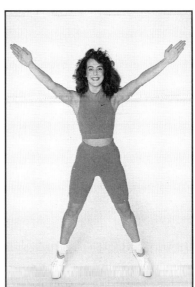

Figure 4.15. (Step 1) Jacks.

Figure 4.16. (Step 2).

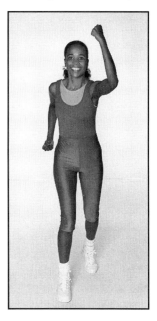

Figure 4.17.
Power pace-walk.

Power Low-Impact Aerobics

Again these are the center-of-gravity lifting, hip-knee-ankle extending moves, followed by the knee-flexion, ankle springing-action moves where one foot is always in contact with the floor, to keep the force of impact low. The time frame can be approximately 5 minutes.

Low-Impact Aerobics Cool-Down

These are the lower intensity moves needed to gradually lower your heart rate. They are still active and rhythmic, using a full range-of-motion, but now are low-level and slower, half-the-tempo moves, like two-foot bouncing and punching (Figure 4.18), and standing upper- and lower-body conditioning moves, like a squat with bicep curls (Figure 4.19). The time frame can be approximately 10 minutes.

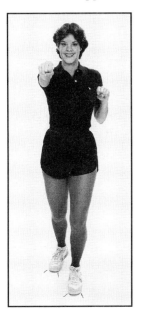

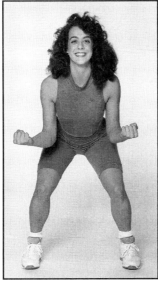

Figure 4.19. Squat and curls.

Figure 4.18. Bouncing.

Post-Aerobic Stretching

Stretching the lower-body muscles to aid blood returning to the heart to prevent blood pooling in the legs is performed by standing static stretches for the hamstrings (Figure 4.20), quadriceps and iliopsoas (Figure 4.21), and calf muscles (Figure 4.22). The time frame can be approximately 3–5 minutes.

— Post-Aerobic Stretching —

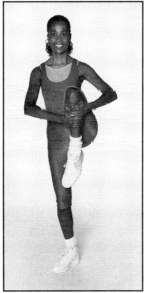

Figure 4.20. Hamstrings.

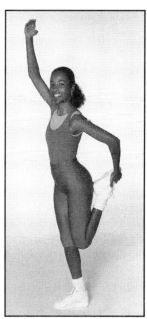

Figure 4.21. Quads.

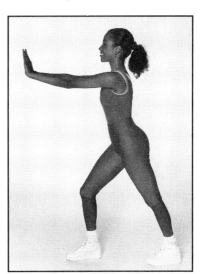

Figure 4.22. Calves.

This concludes the second segment of the workout session called the aerobics segment.

III. Strength Training and Calisthenics Segment

A general strengthening of all of the muscles of the body occurs during vigorous aerobics. However, the optional strength program that is included within an aerobics hour that focuses on the strength development of isolated muscle groups is performed at the end of the aerobics workout but before the final cool-down, flexibility training, and relaxation segment.

The reasoning for this is simple. With an increase in the resistance (weight) that must be applied to any

movement for significant change (i.e., "training") to occur, there is also an increase in the workload that is placed on the heart, lungs, and vascular system. An individual is more readily placed in a breathless "oxygen-debt" state. During the aerobic phase, your goal is *not* to be in a breathless state. You want to be continually working in a breathe-easy state, steadily pacing your intensity.

Strength activities for the chest are push-ups (Figure 4.23) or floor flies (Figures 4.24 and 4.25), short-lever bicep curls for the arms and shoulders (Figure 4.26) and long-lever lateral raises (Figure 4.27), curl-up variations for the abdomen (Figure 4.28), squats for the buttocks (Figure 4.29), leg curls for the thighs (Figures 4.30 and 4.31), alternating ankle flexion and extension for the shins (Figure 4.32), and one-legged calf raises for the calves (Figures 4.33 and 4.34) all represent isolated muscle groups that are strength trained by the associated key exercises shown. These exercises are performed to more quickly define, tone, shape, make more dense, i.e., *thicken* your muscle fibers. It will also allow you to endure longer periods of work during your exercise program and later in your daily work tasks.

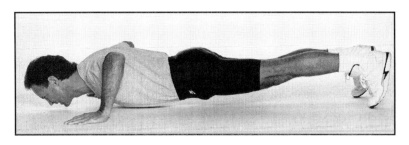

Figure 4.23. CHEST — Push-ups.

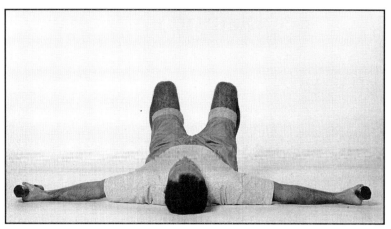

Figure 4.27. CHEST — Floor flies (Step 1).

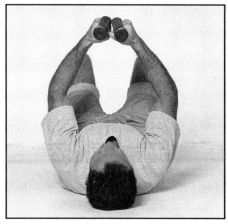

Figure 4.25. CHEST — Floor flies (Step 2).

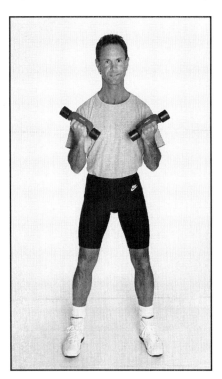

Figure 4.26. ARMS AND SHOULDERS — Short-lever bicep curl.

Figure 4.27. ARMS AND SHOULDERS — Long-lever lateral raise.

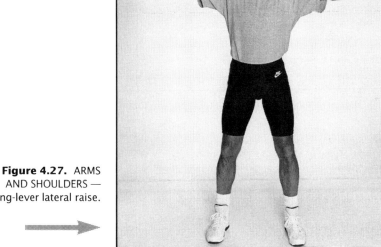

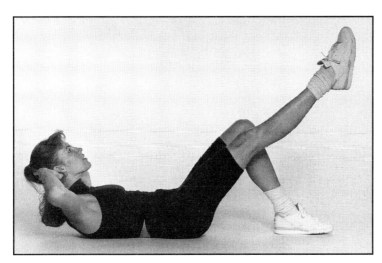

Figure 4.28. ABDOMEN — Curl-up variation.

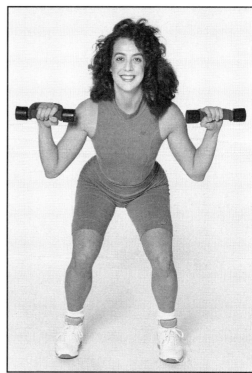

Figure 4.29. BUTTOCKS — Squats.

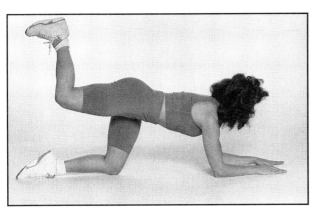

Figure 4.30. THIGH — Leg Curls (Step 1).

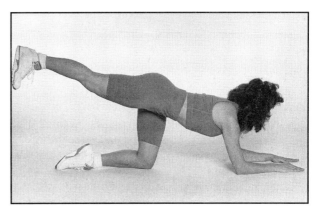

Figure 4.31. THIGH — Leg Curls (Step 2).

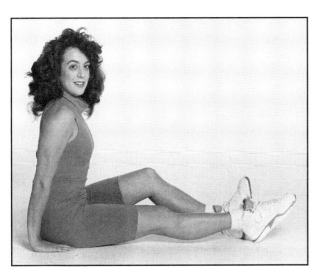

Figure 4.32. SHINS — Alternating ankle flexion and extension.

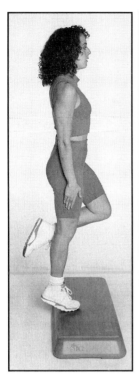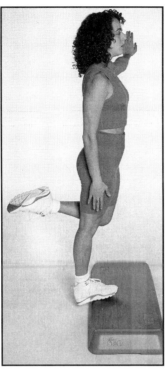

Figure 4.33.   **Figure 4.34.**
CALVES — One-legged calf raise.

Since the focus is now on resistance work, which is best done when the body is thoroughly warmed, the time frame becomes optional and actually according to what you've prioritized time for in your workout session. If possible, plan approximately 10–20 minutes for strength training during aerobics class using the following principles:

► Muscle strengthening exercises should be preceded and followed by stretching exercises that are specific for the muscles that are made to work against resistance. Any muscle group strengthened by exercise should also be regularly stretched to prevent abnormal contraction of resting length.[6]

► Of key importance is the stabilizing of your joints and your spine before beginning each exercise.

► Perform each movement using a smooth, continuous, full range-of-motion action for the joint/muscle group involved, and keep the timing of the movement (usually slow) totally under your control. Ballistic (rapid or jerky) movements increase the risk of injury.

► Proper timing includes taking approximately two seconds to perform the overcoming-resistance-action (concentric) phase, and from two to four

seconds (i.e., at least the same time, or up to twice as long) during the release or lowering (eccentric) phase to return to the starting position of each exercise.[7]

► Exhale during the lifting, overcoming-resistance-action move; inhale during the release or lowering and return. (Exception: during overhead pressing movements, inhale as you lift.)[8]

► Your visualization and self-talk will be of tremendous help here, so plan your concentrated thoughts to accompany your lifting/exhale and lowering/ inhale movements.

► Designing the repetitions of each exercise, and the sets of repetitions that you employ should follow the progressive resistance format. Begin with 1–3 sets of 8–12 repetitions for most exercises. (Exception: for abdominal work, begin your program by performing 2 sets of 15–30 repetitions per set). Select 8–10 exercises that condition the major muscle groups of your body for at least two of your aerobic sessions per week, if you have no other separate strength training program.

► When you become jerky, and are not smooth, continuous, and rhythmical in the move, and are not using the full range-of-motion possible around your joints, you've completed your lower limit possible of that set. Make a record of this number on Chart 14 in the Appendix that will be explained later. This lower limit becomes your baseline to which you attempt to add more repetitions as early as possible.

► It will later be less beneficial if just more repetitions are performed without adding additional resistance. Adding resistance in increasingly greater increments (i.e., from 1–4 pounds if hand weights are used, or thicker rubber if bands/tubing are used) will provide the added resistance you need over the course of your program. However, in the aerobics class setting, don't go over four-pound limit for hand-held weights if this is your choice of resistance equipment.

► Strength training isolated muscle groups is performed on an every other day basis. Your muscles need a day to recover, so don't incorporate a program to strength train with resistance (weights/bands/tubing) daily. An alternative to this program is to perform strength training exercises with resistance (weights/bands/tubing) for the upper half of your body one day, and for the lower half of your body the next day. You are thus alternating the days that the muscles are strength training.

▶ The most efficient way to improve strength is to allow brief rest periods between bouts of vigorous exercises. The time-frame for rest is defined as regaining a normal breathing pattern.

▶ To incorporate variety into your program, try using all of the following forms of resistance:

1) *Your own body (or parts)* lifted and lowered against gravity as the weight resistance used, as in push-ups or curl-ups. (See Figures 4.23 and 4.28). To progressively increase the resistance involved in lifting your body's weight against gravity, a strategically placed free-weight is used (i.e., on the sternum for a curl-up, Figure 7.128, or between the shoulder blades for a push-up, etc.).

2) *Hand-held weights* (not wrist-weights) are used in controlled movement or placed on the body in the key locations to add weight resistance to the body part being lifted and lowered.

3) *Rubber resistance bands* either 9, 12 or 16 inches long, in widths of 1/4–1½ inches can be used. The length and width is selected according to whether it is an upper or lower body exercise, and your current strength fitness level in the muscle group being trained.

4) *Rubber resistance tubing*, approximately 3–4½ feet long so that you can adjust it according to your height in a range of light to heavy thickness that you select according to your current level of strength fitness.

5) You may also combine all the above, using a step-bench in a level position, or in the gravity-assisted incline or decline positions. You will begin to realize from the exercises shown in Chapter 7 that the possibilities for variety in your strength training segment are fun, exciting, inexpensive, and absolutely unlimited!

Options number 3, 4, and 5 are shown in Figure 4.35. Following are the principles for using these unique pieces of equipment.

Using Resistance Bands and Tubing

The general directions for using either resistance bands or tubing are:

▶ Select bands and tubing based on your fitness level.

▶ Always inspect the bands and tubing before each use for nicks and tears that may arise from continued use.

▶ Never, under any circumstances, should you tie pieces of band and tubing together.

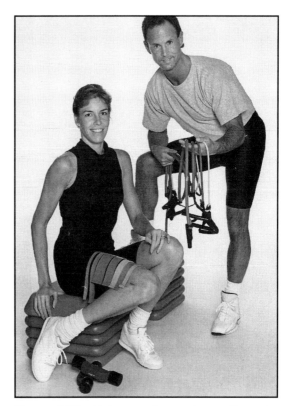

Figure 4.35. Various equipment to use for resistance when exercising.

▶ Always exhibit proper body alignment and posture while exercising, as shown in the following figures.

▶ Keep your face turned slightly away from the direction of movement, to assure safety.

▶ Always anchor the band between one hand and the thigh, hip, side or shoulder, depending on the movement, while performing single limb upper body movements.

▶ Always anchor the tubing under the ball of one foot or both feet, depending on your level of fitness and the desired amount of tension you wish to create.

▶ Always control the bands and tubing, especially during the return phase of the movement. Do not let them control you.

▶ Perform 8–10 repetitions of each exercise. When one arm or leg is used, switch sides so the same muscle group is worked an equal number of repetitions on the opposite side of the body. Be sure to work all muscular groups with equal intensity and repetitions at each session, to avoid muscular imbalance.[9]

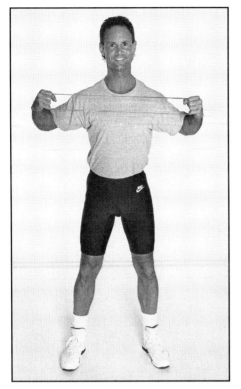

Using resistance bands for the upper body —
deltoid press-away and lower body — leg extension
for the quadriceps

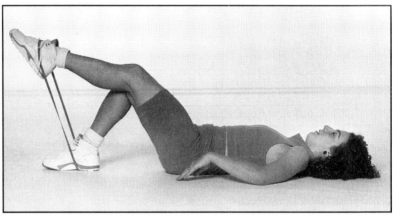

Figure 4.36.   **Figure 4.37.**

Bands

Bands are available in a variety of sizes to vary the intensity of your workout.[10] Suggested sizes:

▶ **Beginner**

3/8" upper body (pink) or (light blue)
3/8" or 5/8" lower body

▶ **Intermediate**

5/8" upper body (light blue)
5/8" lower body

▶ **Advanced**

3/4" upper body (dark blue)
3/4" lower body

Tubing

Tubing is also available in a variety of sizes to vary the intensity of your workout.[11] Suggested sizes:

▶ **Beginner**

Very Light and Light Tubing (yellow or green)

▶ **Intermediate**

Light and Medium Tubing (green or red)

▶ **Advanced**

Heavy Tubing (blue)

All of the tubing exercises described in Chapter 7 are designed for the beginner and intermediate exerciser. This means one foot will always be placed on the center of the tubing to create resistance. You can use the other foot to anchor the tubing if you prefer. Participants who want to create more resistance, simply stand on the tubing with both feet. The wider you spread your feet, the more resistance you will create (Figures 4.38–4.40).[12]

The Bench-Step and Tubing Exercises

There are also a variety of exercises presented in Chapter 7 using the tubing in combination with the bench-step, for either just weight training, or for an interval aerobics/strength training workout. The key to the latter workout is incorporating one minute intervals of tubing exercises using the bench, with the body pressed into a "bent-knees" position on the action of the exercise. This position helps to keep the heart rate in the training zone, during strength training and provides another safe, unique variety of exercises in your aerobics programming.

Monitor and Chart Your Progress

On Chart 14 in the Appendix entitled, "Strength Training with Bands, Tubing, Light 1–4 lb. Weights, and Tubing with The Bench," record the exercises you perform, plus the number of sets, repetitions and

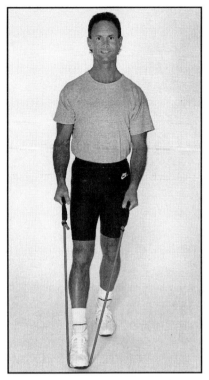

Figure 4.38. BEGINNER — Place 1 foot on tubing.

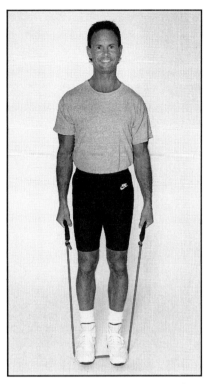

Figure 4.39. INTERMEDIATE — Place both feet on tubing.

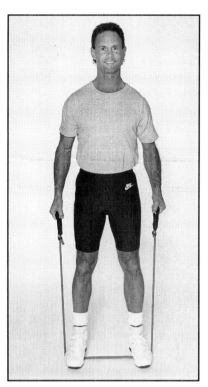

Figure 4.40. ADVANCED — Spread feet on tubing.

the type and amount of resistance you used with each exercise. Charting your progress gives you a visual blueprint for success, adherence, and is a means of continual motivation!

Summary

Finally, just remember to begin your program slowly, methodically, and in absolute control of the amount of resistance or weights you are using. Strength-fitness training to more fully develop muscle strength and endurance is a long-term project [13] calling for a dedicated personal commitment of many hours, just as the programs of stretching for flexibility improvement, and aerobics for aerobic capacity improvement are. All fitness programs are for life.

IV. Cool-Down, Flexibility Training and Relaxation

Cool Down is Gradual

The purpose of a planned cool-down portion of your hour is to give your body time to re-adjust back to the pre-activity state in which you began. This will ease the gradual process of returning the large quantity of blood that is now in your working muscles, primarily in your arms and legs, back toward your head and trunk, brain and other vital organs. An abrupt stopping of a highly strenuous activity session may cause the blood (primarily in your legs) to "pool" or stay in the extremities. This will occur because the veins of the legs are not being forcefully squeezed now by strenuously working leg muscles.

The result of this "pooling" can cause cramping, nausea, dizziness, and fainting since the needed quantity of oxygen and blood is not being delivered to the brain and other vital organs. So do not forget this very important last phase.

Your ability to recover from exertion will usually determine how long of a cool-down you will need to include. A minimum of five to ten minutes is essential, however, for two reasons:

▶ To curtail profuse sweating.

▶ To lower the heart rate to below 120 beats per minutes.

These are two visible signs to monitor and achieve before concluding your exercise hour.

You'll begin your cooling down process with a complete slowing down of all large muscle activity. Tapering off your activity level can be performed in various ways, such as slow tempoed aerobics moves (Figure 4.41), slow-paced walking, etc. This segment begins the transition between the vigorous activity

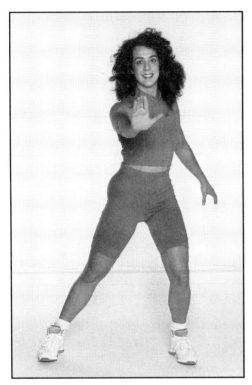

Figure 4.41. Cool-down with slow-tempoed aerobics moves.

you've just completed, and the flexibility training and relaxation that you perform last.

Flexibility Training

Flexibility training, or *stretching*, is widely accepted as an effective means of increasing joint mobility, improving exercise performance and reducing injuries.[14] Proper technique is essential, for the risks of injury may be significant if stretches are incorrectly performed.

Flexibility refers to the range-of-motion of a certain joint and its corresponding muscle groups. It is genetically influenced and highly specific and varies from joint to joint within an individual. Muscle, when repeatedly stretched, can be lengthened by approximately 20 percent,[15] while tendons can increase in length only about 2 to 3 percent.

Stretching programs follow the principle Specific Adaptation to Imposed Demands (SAID), which states that an individual must slowly and progressively stretch the soft tissues around a joint to and slightly beyond the point of limitation, but not to the point of tearing.

Two Methods of Stretching

At present, the two most widely accepted methods of stretching for improving flexibility are static and Proprioceptive Neuromuscular Facilitatory (PNF) techniques. Both techniques follow the philosophy that flexibility is increased and risk of injury is prevented when the muscle being stretched is as relaxed as possible.

Static Stretching is slow, active stretching, with the position held at the joint extremes. The technique for executing stretching efficiently and safely is to gently ease into a controlled, stretched position and hold it as you gently press (Figure 4.42). You push or press to the point of tightness, "stretch pull" (not a pain, but a tight feeling) so that you feel the muscle working. You then continue to stretch a little beyond this point, without any motion. Mentally, then, you relax your mind and hold the position for approximately 15 seconds, allowing the muscle to also relax and feel heavier.[16] Continue to relax and slowly withdraw the stretch. Performing the same stretching on the opposite side of your body always follows.

At present, static stretching is considered to be one of the most effective methods of increasing flexibility and research has shown that significant gains can be achieved with a training program of static stretching exercises. This type of continuous, long stretching produces greater flexibility with less possibility of injury, probably because it stretches the muscles under controlled conditions.

PNF Stretching techniques, where muscles are progressively stretched with intermittent isometric contractions, are also a very effective method of increasing flexibility and are used, like static stretches, when the muscles are warm. Two of the most commonly used modified PNF stretches are:

▶ Contract-relax technique: In phase one, a five- to six-second maximum voluntary contraction in the muscle to be stretched is performed by the

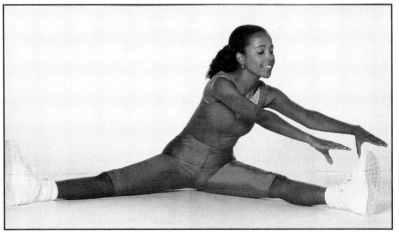

Figure 4.42. Static stretching.

exerciser. The contraction is isometric, since any motion is resisted. In phase two, the previously contracted muscle is relaxed, then stretched.

▶ Agonist contract-relax technique: In phase one, the exerciser maximally contracts the muscle opposite the muscle to be stretched against resistance (a partner, the floor, or other immovable object) for five to six seconds. In phase two, the agonist muscle is relaxed and the antagonist muscle stretched.[17]

An example of a forward PNF contract-relax exercise for the hamstrings and spinal extensors is shown in Figure 4.43 and is performed with a partner's assistance. The position and actions are detailed.

▶ *Position:* In a modified hurdler stretch position, the performing partner leans forward to the point of limitation while keeping the back straight and the toes of the extended leg facing upward to correctly stretch the hamstrings.

▶ *Action*: To begin the action, the performer pushes her back against the partner (contracting the spinal extensors) and pushes the extended leg against the floor (contracting the hamstrings) for a six-second isometric contraction. The partner gently, but firmly, resists any movement.

▶ *Action*: After releasing the contraction, the performer stretches to a new point of limitation, holding a static stretch for 12 seconds, or more, while the partner maintains a very light pressure on the performer's back.

Research has shown both static and PNF techniques for stretching are effective. Both techniques can be successfully used to enhance one's flexibility.

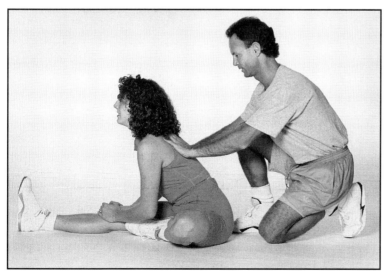

Figure 4.43. Forward PNF contract-relax stretching.

Relaxation

Relaxation techniques complete your total physical fitness hour and can be incorporated first during the stretching phase (Figure 4.44), to realize greater flexibility gains, and continued when stretching is completed, when there is an absence of muscle tension established throughout the body.

When mental relaxation is initiated during the final stretching phase of the workout hour, there are three key factors the participant will focus on:

▶ Your mental images that are being constructed.

▶ Your self-talk accompanying each stretch and release (or contract-relax, according to which technique you use).

▶ The mechanics of your breathing pattern.

It is usually quite interesting to realize that to become highly motivated early on and then to relax at the end requires a person to key into the same set of internal resources. The only difference between these two extremes is *how* you use these resources.

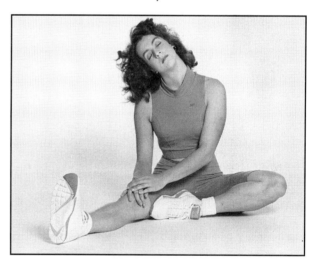

Figure 4.44. Combining relaxation with stretching segment.

Static Stretching with Relaxation

The mental images made for relaxation initiated during the final stretching phase matches the self-talk that accompanies it. The muscles being isolated and stretched are pictured and affirmed as becoming "wider, and longer, and warmer, and heavier."

Your breathing pattern is sequenced with these pictures and affirmations. An

8-count deep breath starts the whole procedure and is initiated from deep down in the diaphragm area and inhaled through your nose. This deep breath is held several seconds (up to eight). As you slowly exhale through your pursed lips, you formulate the pictures and affirmations: "wider-longer-warmer-heavier" — "wider longer warmer-heavier." Take about 16 seconds to slowly exhale and static stretch with these pictures and affirmations. Finally, as the stretch is slowly released and the muscle relaxed, another deep 8-count inhalation begins.

To match pictures and affirmations with the PNF stretching, mentally take apart the muscular actions that are transpiring and the time-frame suggested for each portion to take. The exhalation breathing is performed during the contractions.

Program Segments In Review

The basic principles for the four key segments of an aerobics program workout session have been established with further detail given on the components within each segment. Outlined, they include:

Segment I — The Warm-Up
▶ Active, rhythmic, limbering moves
▶ Slow, standing, static stretching.
▶ Proper breathing techniques throughout.

Segment II — Aerobics
▶ Low impact cardiovascular warm-up.
▶ Power low impact with plyometrics.
▶ High and low impact.
▶ Power low impact with plyometrics.
▶ Low impact cool down.
▶ Post-aerobic stretching.

Segment III — Strength Training and Calisthenics
▶ Focusing on isolated muscle groups — chest, arms, abdominals, buttocks, thighs, shins and calves.
▶ Adding free weights, assistance bands and tubing, and bench exercises.

Segment IV — Cool Down, Flexibility Improvement, and Relaxation Techniques
▶ Gradual cool-down moves.
▶ Flexibility training using static and PNF stretching.
▶ Relaxation techniques during stretching.

Following an aerobics program such as this will provide you with a fun, safe, efficient and complete workout session. If this type of total physical fitness program is prioritized into your schedule for a minimum of three days per week, you will have found an excellent means of initially obtaining and then maintaining, your fitness for a lifetime.

ENJOYMENT THROUGH AEROBIC VARIETIES

Introducing Bench/Step Training

Bench/Step training, or "step training", is currently the hottest aerobic trend of the 1990's and is sweeping the aerobics fitness industry with a new burst of enthusiasm! It is a relatively unexplored new training modality with little research to date, so all the related common problems and injuries have not yet been fully assessed. To date the following information and guidelines have been presented by various researchers promoting the activity, and companies promoting products to use with the activity.[18, 19, 20, 21, 22]

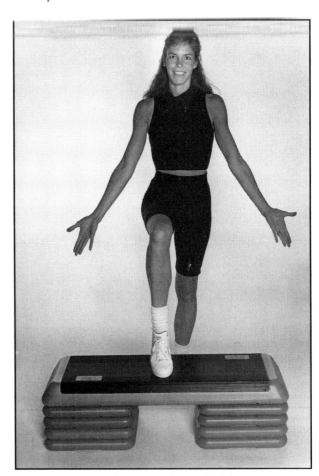

Figure 4.45. Introducing Bench-Step Training.

Definitions, Advantages and Benefits

Step training is an exercise activity that involves stepping up and down on a platform or bench with a variety of upper torso movements added for further challenge. It enjoys a variety of names: bench or step aerobics, bench or step training, bench stepping, and stepping are just a few, and all refer to the same activity.

The benefits are many. The key advantage to a step training program is that it is primarily a *high intensity activity* used to promote cardiorespiratory fitness, but *with low impact* for safety concerns, since a vast majority of all the moves can involve one foot supporting your weight, either on the bench platform, or on the floor. Other benefits include the following:

▶ It's a terrific conditioning workout for the muscles of the legs, hips, and buttocks.

▶ Upper torso movements may provide conditioning work for muscles or arms, shoulders, chest and back and therefore a balanced and complete workout that strengthens and tones the entire body. This becomes especially apparent later when and if you advance to using 1–4 lb. light hand weights in a controlled manner, in conjunction with your stepping moves.

▶ As an effective cardiovascular workout, it has the aerobics benefits equal to running 7 mph, and yet has the potentially low-impact equivalence of walking at a 3 mph pace.[23]

▶ This workout is unique in its aerobics class versatility. The basic moves are simple and by introducing various step patterns, all levels of participants can be simultaneously challenged. Regardless of sex or age, individuals can work at their own fitness level simply by doing less (or more) arm gestures, by adjusting the height of the bench, and by choosing to add or omit hand weights.

Choosing Your Bench Height

When choosing a bench height, consider each of the following factors:

▶ As a beginner or novice, who has not exercised regularly, or has limited coordination, or no experience in step training, you should select a 4" to 6" bench initially. (For the 12" bench shown in Figure 4.45, this represents the basic 4" platform, and at most *one* 2" support block on each end.)

▶ As an intermediate, or regular step trainer with a "physically fit" level of cardiorespiratory fitness, choose an 8"–10" step. (For the bench shown in Figure 4.45, an 8" bench equals the platform and two 2" support blocks. For a 10" bench, add three 2" support blocks).

▶ As an advanced, or skilled regular step trainer with a high level of cardiovascular fitness, choose a 10"–12" step. (For the bench in Figure 4.45, the platform plus a maximum of 4 support blocks on each end).

▶ Participant height and leg length may dictate that a taller individual may prefer a bench step of 8"–12".

▶ Regardless of level of fitness or experience, do not select a step height that allows the knee to exceed 90 degrees of flexion (Figure 4.46) when the knee is weight bearing.

An optional test for bench height is shown in Figure 4.47. Place one foot flat on top of the bench; allow a 3" drop from the hip to knee for safe movement up to the top of the bench.

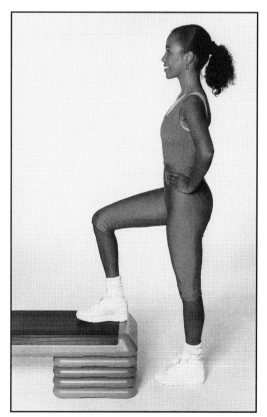

Figure 4.46. Standard guideline is to not exceed a 90 degree knee angle as participant steps up on the bench and bears weight.

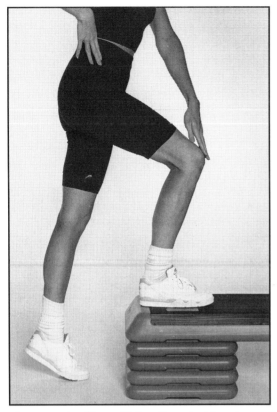

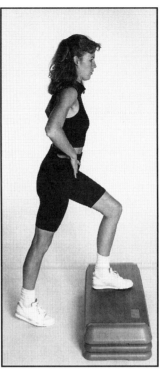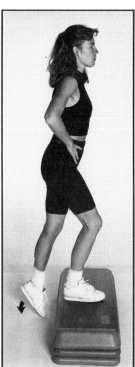

Figure 4.48.   **Figure 4.49.**
Proper technique for stepping up and stepping down.

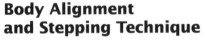

Figure 4.47. Allow a 3" drop from the hip to knee.

Body Alignment and Stepping Technique

Good posture is required for a safe, injury-free workout. Proper alignment and stepping technique include:

▶ Keep your back straight, head and chest up, shoulders back, abdomen tight and buttocks tucked under hips, with eyes on the platform. (Figure 4.48)

▶ As much as possible, keep your shoulders aligned over your hips. Lean forward with the whole body. Don't bend from the hips or round the shoulders and lean forward or backward.

▶ Step up lightly, making sure the whole foot lands on the platform, with the heel bearing your weight.

▶ Keep your knees aligned over your feet when they're pulling your body weight onto the platform.

▶ At the top, straighten your legs but don't lock your knees — keep them "soft."

▶ As you step down, stay close to the platform. Land on the ball of the foot, (Figure 4.49) then bring the heel down onto the floor, before taking the next step.

Step Technique Progression

Beginners should start on a 4" bench, using no weights at a moderate tempo for no more than 10 minutes per session.[24] As you progress in skill and fitness level, the length of time stepping can be increased. When you can easily complete an entire session, the platform height can be raised, the music tempo increased, the arms can be used through a wider range-of-motion, and 1 to 4 lb. hand weights can be added.

However, only one variable should be changed during a session. Don't increase platform height and add weights at the same time. Increasing several variables at the same time doesn't allow your body time to adequately adapt to these additional changes and stressors.

Start with your hands on your hips and concentrate on your feet and legs as your first priority. Once you've become proficient with the basic footwork skills and your fitness level has improved, increase the intensity of your program through your arm movements. This can include controlled complicated arm gestures *or* the use of hand weights.

The arm movements used with or without weights, are those taken from strength training programs that safely use long- and short-lever moves in a full range-of-motion action. All arm movements, however, must move with the step pattern. This means arms go forward when stepping on the bench, back when stepping off, and up on a propulsion move. Think to use muscle more than momentum (i.e. control) and you will keep it a safer workout.

A Few Precautions:

▶ Avoid excessive arm movements over your head.

▶ Maintain appropriate speed for safe and effective movement.

▶ Repeated foot impact without variation is potentially harmful; do not perform not more than 8 counts (4 repeaters) on one leg at a time.

▶ Do not pivot or twist the knee on the weight-bearing leg.

▶ Do not step up or down with your back towards the platform.

▶ If you are pregnant, check with your doctor before starting this program. If you are cleared by your doctor, make certain that you keep your heart rate at 23 beats or below for a 10 second count. It is recommended a step height of no more than six inches be used during pregnancy.

▶ If you feel faint or dizzy or if any exercise causes pain or severe discomfort, stop the exercise immediately but continue to move around.

▶ No more than one person should perform on a bench at a time.

▶ For the bench shown in Figure 4.45, do not use more than four support blocks on each end of the platform.

Adding Hand-Held Weights to Stepping

The benefits of using 1–4 lb. hand-held weights in a step-training program includes the fact that you can increase both exercise intensity for continual cardiovascular fitness gains, and muscular strength and tonus, especially in the upper torso with the use of weights.

The low impact nature of step training, along with controlled stepping patterns performed at a moderate tempo make it possible to safely use hand held weights[26], provided the following safety precautions and those previously mentioned, are followed.

1. Only when participants are proficient at step training and when they have achieved an intermediate level of fitness should hand weights be added, using one or two pound weights only (Figure 4.50).

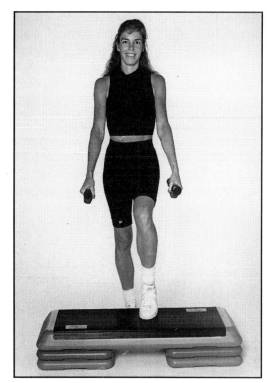

Figure 4.50.

2. Hand weights should *not* be used by those who
   ▶ Have high blood pressure.
   ▶ Have a history of coronary disease.
   ▶ Suffer from low back pain.
   ▶ Have arthritis.
   ▶ Have other chronic or temporary orthopedic problems.
   ▶ Are past the first trimester of pregnancy.
   ▶ Are significantly overweight.

3. When you begin using light weights, use them for just one routine per session and gradually build up your endurance. Remember this key thought: start low and go slow.

4. Begin by using slow, small ranges-of-motion with short-lever, non-rotational arm movements, and never use flinging or uncontrolled movements.

5. Avoid overuse of maintaining arms at or above shoulder level for extended periods of time (i.e., overuse of tendons that stabilize the shoulder joint and unnecessary blood pressure elevation.)

6. Avoid full-arm extension moves, in short counts of music time.

7. Avoid using weights while performing propulsion steps.

8. Feel free to put weights down during your workout at any time. Place them safely under your bench, or somewhere you'll not accidentally step on them.

Adjusting Your Intensity

To decrease or increase your heart rate pulse, try the following measures:

To Decrease

1. No weights.
2. Keep hands on hips.
3. Lower bench height.
4. Perform movements only on floor.
5. Slow music tempo.

To Increase

1. Larger range-of-motion arm movements.
2. Add 2" support blocks to bench height.
3. Add use of 1–4 lb. hand-held weights.
4. Increase music tempo.

STEP TRAINING SUMMARY

There are many advantages and benefits to incorporating a bench step training program in your lifetime aerobics fitness plan. The key is that it is a high intensity exercise that sustains the training zone heart-rate needed for the cardiorespiratory training effect to occur. Yet it is low-impact and safe since one foot remains on the bench or the ground. Maintaining the safe precautions of selecting the correct bench height, good body positioning and alignment, variety in technique so over-use does not occur, and following the extensive guidelines for safely incorporating arm gestures and adding weights, all work together to establish an exciting new modality variety of aerobics training. Chapter 7 presents the details of techniques to use.

ANOTHER AEROBICS OPTION: PACE-WALKING

Easiest of all aerobic options is probably this one since it can be done anywhere with no need for equipment or other's direction. It takes three times as long to get the same aerobic benefit from walking as from running[27], so *time* is a key factor when planning variety. Walking, incidentally, is action that takes 14 minutes or longer per mile as compared to jogging at 9–12 minutes per mile or running at under 9 minutes per mile.[28] Important points for

pace-walking in regards to principles and techniques are:

▶ Wear a supportive walking or running shoe and loose comfortable clothing.

▶ Walk with the heel of the shoe contacting the ground first (Figure 4.51), with a rolling action forward, continue through the ball of the foot. Eliminate any tendency for a bobbing, up and down motion.

▶ Arms are held in a long-lever (relaxed-elbow) position, with a forward and backward controlled swinging motion to involve upper torso conditioning also.

▶ If weights are used, follow all of the guidelines given earlier for using hand-held weights with special attention to controlling your arm motions. Use very light weights if any are used at all.

▶ Posture is kept erect at all times with a relaxed lower back. Swing your hips freely forward and backward. Enjoy an easy, continuous breathing pattern.

▶ Follow all the aforementioned guidelines for aerobics programming, including an adequate warm-up and cool-down.

A Level I 10-Week Walking Program is shown on Table 4.1. Remember to

1. warm-up and cool-down, and
2. walk briskly for at least 45 minutes, 3 to 5 times per week to achieve maximum aerobic benefit from this program.[29]

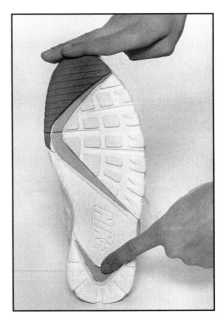

Figure 4.51. Walk with the heel of the shoe contacting the ground first.

TABLE 4.1   Level I — Walking Only*

Week	Session	Warm Up	Exercise	Warm Down	Goal (Distance)
1	1	yes	15-20'	yes	0.5 to 0.8 mi.
	2	yes	15-20'	yes	0.9 to 1.0 mi.
	3	yes	20'	yes	0.9 to 1.0 mi.
2	4	yes	20'	yes	0.9 to 1.0 mi.
	5	yes	24'	yes	1.1 to 1.2 mi.
	6	yes	24'	yes	1.1 to 1.2 mi.
3	7	yes	28'	yes	1.3 to 1.4 mi.
	8	yes	28'	yes	1.3 to 1.4 mi.
	9	yes	32'	yes	1.4 to 1.6 mi.
4	10	yes	32'	yes	1.4 to 1.6 mi.
	11	yes	36'	yes	1.7 to 1.8 mi.
	12	yes	36'	yes	1.7 to 1.8 mi.
5	13	yes	40'	yes	1.9 to 2.0 mi.
	14	yes	40'	yes	1.9 to 2.0 mi.
	15	yes	44'	yes	2.1 to 2.2 mi.
6	16	yes	48'	yes	2.3 to 2.4 mi.
	17	yes	48'	yes	2.3 to 2.4 mi.
	18	yes	48'	yes	2.3 to 2.4 mi.
7	19	yes	52'	yes	2.5 to 2.6 mi.
	20	yes	52'	yes	2.5 to 2.6 mi.
	21	yes	56'	yes	2.7 to 2.8 mi.
8	22	yes	56'	yes	2.7 to 2.8 mi.
	23	yes	60'	yes	2.9 to 3.0 mi.
	24	yes	60'	yes	2.9 to 3.0 mi.
9	25	yes	58'	yes	3.0 mi.
	26	yes	58'	yes	3.0 mi.
	27	yes	56'	yes	3.0 mi.
10	28	yes	56'	yes	3.0 mi.
	29	yes	54'	yes	3.0 mi.
	30	yes	54'	yes	3.0 mi.

*Program written by Dr. Richard Bowers, ACSM certified Program Director

ANOTHER OPTION: JUMPING ROPE

Rope jumping is a very strenuous activity that uses approximately three times more energy than leisure walking. Thus, such an impact activity is not suited for everyone. Inactive individuals or those with joint or back problems should not participate in this form of aerobics. Others with exercise experience should have no problem.

Principles to consider are the following:

▶ For jumping rope you need a rope of correct length, and preferably a giving surface upon which to jump. The correct length of rope is for it to reach your armpits (Figure 4.52) when held down tightly under your feet with a few extra inches, or a handle, with which to hold the rope comfortably. If no handles are present, tape the

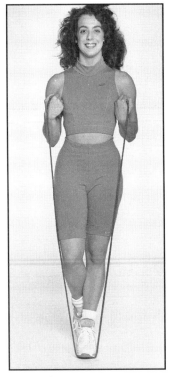

Figure 4.52. Selecting correct length of rope.

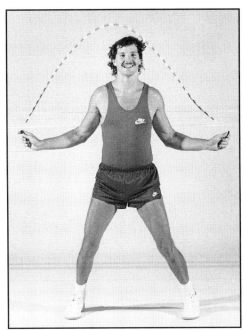

Figure 4.53.

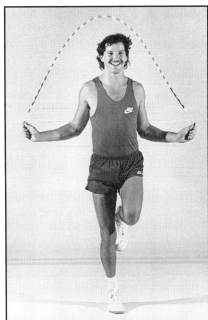

Figure 4.54.

ends or tie knots at the ends to help prevent fraying. There are a variety of jump ropes on the market, including beaded licorice, leather and cotton ropes. Beaded ropes and leather ropes are the best choice. Licorice (plastic) get tangled more frequently and cotton ropes are rather difficult to use because they are so light-weight.

▶ When you warm up, be sure to static stretch all the muscles of the leg with special attention to the calf, heel cord, and shin areas.

▶ The aerobics segment can begin with six minutes and as you progress, can lead up to a 20 minute workout.

▶ Restrict continuous jumping to one minute intervals at 120–140 revolutions per minute which is a moderate pace. Alternating one-minute segments with non-jumping low-impact aerobics such as marching or power walking. Music should range from 120–140 beats per minute also, to assist in timing and rhythm.

▶ Jumping techniques include jumping low with "soft" knees for efficiency and only high enough to clear the rope (less than one inch).

▶ Use rate of perceived exertion for monitoring your intensity because it will allow you to have a minute-to-minute monitoring of how you feel.

▶ Be sure to provide both a 5–10 minute cool down which includes non-jumping low-impact

moves, and flexibility and relaxation for 5 minutes in which static stretching for the leg muscles used, are again performed.[30]

Try a variety of rope-jumping skills (Figures 4.53 and 4.54):

1) One foot and then the other. If you jump on only one foot, don't do more than four repetitions on the same foot. Alternate immediately to the other foot for the same number of steps.

2) Two feet at a time.

3) Jump with arm/rope crossed, followed by a one-foot or two-foot jump.

4) Hopscotch jump, two-foot jump stride, one-foot jump, two-foot jump stride, alternate one-foot jump.

MONITOR AND CHART YOUR PROGRESS

It is always enjoyable to experience becoming and maintaining progress towards total physical fitness. Take time immediately after each exercise session to record your progress and gains in a journal. Be sure to record any set-backs also. It will give you a visual blueprint on how you are successfully accomplishing a variety of short-term goals, and how you can duplicate it in the future. Include the following type of entries: today's date, exercise varieties used, time duration, short-term goal set, new achievement today, and your thoughts and feelings.

Chapter 5

Special Concerns — Problems & Solutions!

The enjoyment found in a new activity can bring long-lasting benefits to your total wellness and vitality. Positive gains can constantly be achieved when the principles for safe, efficient movement are followed. There is, however, an element of risk associated with all physical activities that is apparent and must be addressed. When proper preventative measures are taken, problems or injuries can be avoided. The following concerns are detailed in order to increase your awareness regarding the more common program-related problems that you may incur. Understanding prevention before the occurrence is the key to a safe program.

GRADUAL, SENSIBLE — DON'T OVERDO IT!

It takes a planned self-discipline to become and stay physically fit, but the dividends of wellness and vitality are well worth it.

Progress gradually and sensibly in your sessions. Remember to warm up and cool down and to progress from easy to advanced both in the stretches and in the aerobic combinations. Learn to read your body signs. You're going to perspire and you're going to tire *a little*, but keep performing. However, you do not need to perform to the point of exhaustion. Know that with an effective aerobics program you may encounter some initial, slight, temporary discomfort, so be sensible about pacing yourself. For example, after engaging in several aerobic exercise movements or a complete step training routine, you may be short of breath, but this should subside within minutes after the activity. If it doesn't subside,

you've worked too hard. If you are unsure about a particular discomfort or pain, ask a reliable person (such as your doctor) before you continue with the activity.

DEFINITE SIGNS OF OVEREXERTION

While monitoring your pulse helps you determine how hard to exercise your body, you also need to be aware of your own bodily signs. Signs of overexertion are:

▶ Severe breathlessness.

▶ Poor heart rate response (continually monitoring too high an exercising heart rate that does not significantly drop after one minute of recovery or final heart rate not below 120 beats per minute after five minutes of cool-down).

▶ Undue fatigue during exercise and inability to recover from a workout later in the day.

▶ Inability to sleep at night.

▶ Persistent severe muscle soreness. (The type of muscle soreness to guard against is not the immediate type but that which becomes apparent after twenty-four to forty-eight hours.

▶ Nausea, feeling faint, dizziness.

▶ Tightness or pains in the chest.

These symptoms do not mean that you should not exercise; rather, they suggest performing a reduced level of activity until you develop the capacity to handle more intense workouts. It is important to embark on an exercise program cautiously and to *increase gradually* the frequency, the intensity, and/or the time duration of your program.

If you have any of these symptoms, ease down to a slow walk, sit down with your head between your knees, or lie down on your back and elevate your feet. This will help the blood move to your head more easily and carry the needed oxygen to your brain. If any of these symptoms last longer than a brief period of time, contact your doctor.

Note
Seek medical advice immediately and before the next exercise session if any of the following symptoms occur:

1 *Abnormal heart action*
   ▶ Pulse becoming irregular.
   ▶ Fluttering, jumping, or palpitations in chest or throat.
   ▶ Sudden burst of rapid heartbeats.
   ▶ Sudden, very slow pulse when a moment before it had been on target (immediate or delayed).

2 *Pain or pressure in the center of the chest or the arm or throat precipitated by exercise or following exercise (immediate or delayed).*

3 *Dizziness, light-headedness, sudden incoordination, confusion, cold sweat, glassy stare, pallor, blueness, or fainting (immediate).*

Do not try to cool down. Stop exercise and lie down with your feet elevated, or put your head down between your legs until the symptoms pass.[1]

CONSIDER THE VARIABLES

There are numerous variables to be considered and planned for when engaging in an aerobics program, such as when illness, infection or injury is present; if you have not exercised for a while; location and environment; and shoe selection.

When Illness, Infection, or Injury is Present

The presence of illness, infection, or injury will show up in your "thermometer" of fitness — your pulse. It will be higher at rest and will escalate to the training zone with less than your usual effort. So take it easy and decide whether to mentally "walk"

through your program to maintain your discipline of exercising, or to just curtail exercise until you're completely well again.

Missing A While?

Return to aerobics slowly. If for any reason you miss activity several times, you will need to start more cautiously as though beginning a new program. For example, you may have a bout of flu and are unable to exercise for a week. When you are able to exercise again, do *not* plan to start where you left off. You will need to return cautiously to the fitness level that you were at before the illness. Dr. Lenore Zohlman, a leading cardiologist in the United States, has stated that after just five weeks you will lose approximately half of your fitness program gains if you discontinue your program totally. And, after ten weeks of no aerobic activity, you will have lost most of the fitness gains that you experienced.[2] So realize this physiological phenomenon and return slowly and systematically whenever a circumstance curtails your program.

Choose the Best Location & Environment

Select a convenient and physiologically safe location for your program. Choose a wood-based floor or an area carpeted with flat nap and thick padding. (Carpeted surfaces tend to make lateral moves and turns risky, however.) Try not to exercise on concrete, since there is no "give" or buoyancy to it. Concrete adds unnecessary stress on your legs and feet.

"A resilient floor should be selected for exercise that involves repeated foot impacts. If such a surface is not available, the exercise routines should be modified to ensure that the feet remain close to the floor throughout the program."[3] This means you should perform only low-impact exercises.

If there is a high relative humidity combined with a temperature of 85° room or outside temperature, curtail your aerobic dance-exercise or step-training programs. Seek out another option like aerobic swimming in a cool-air environment.

For aerobic exercise, it doesn't matter how cold the environment is, as long as you thoroughly protect yourself, especially your air passages (at 40° and below, cover your air passages). It does matter how *hot* the temperature is, however. Heat stress injuries can occur when caution is abandoned.

Shoe Selection

Wearing proper shoes is one of your major concerns. When you jump or run, you place three to six times more force on your feet than when you are stationary. If you weigh 125 pounds, this means that you are placing 375 to 750 pounds of pressure on your feet with each jump or run. Your body can withstand the stress of exercise better if this extra pressure is "shock absorbed" by the shoe you wear, or the giving quality of the surface upon which you move. Select a shoe that totally supports your foot for the exercise modality you choose to engage in regularly. Read the following criteria, and also refer to Table 5.1 for personalizing your shoe selection.

▶ Inquire about midsole composition. For durability and performance select shoes made from either compression-molded ethyl vinyl acetate (EVA) or polyurethane.

▶ Do not be afraid to stay with the same brand and model of shoe you are currently replacing.

▶ Make a commitment that you will not be forced or pressured into buying a shoe that does not feel comfortable.

▶ Generally, a single pair of shoes worn at least four days per week for any fitness-related activity should be replaced every four months. If the shoes have a polyurethane midsole, the wear may be extended up to six months. If they have a standard, open-cell, EVA midsole, they may last only three months.

▶ Examine the inside of the shoe as well as the insole. Shoes with removable insoles are preferable because they tend to be better cushioned and allow the fit of a custom foot orthotic, if needed.[4]

▶ Nylon uppers are cooler than leather uppers. If an all-leather shoe is preferred, be sure ventilation holes are present on the top and sides. Extra design leather or suede along the ball-edge of the foot area (toes) provides for a longer shoe life.

▶ The sole of the shoe should have a relatively smooth tread[6] and should be of white rubber, designed for aerobic dance-exercise or court use. Jogging shoes with black rubber soles, designed

---

TABLE 5.1   Personalizing Your Shoe Selection[5]

IF YOU:	PICK A SHOE THAT:
are heavier or taller	has a firm, dense midsole, like polyurethane (PU).
are lilghter or smaller	has a softer midsole, like compression-molded ethyl vinyl acetate (EVA).
have a high arch	is well cushioned and soft.
have a flexible arch or flat foot	is firm and has motion-control features.

IF YOU HAVE HAD:	PICK A SHOE THAT:
stress fractures	is cushioned in the midsole and insole.
plantar fasciitis	is flexible, and has a well-contoured insole with a prominent arch support.
ankle sprains	has a firm PU midsole with a 3/4-high reinforced upper.
shin splints	has an elevated heel, plenty of cushion, and a contoured arch insole.
knee problems	has a firm sole with lateral reinforcement in the upper.

IF YOU REGULARLY PARTICIPATE IN:	YOU NEED:
aerobics/dance exercise only	an aerobic-dance shoe or a cross trainer. If you have had arch or heel problems, choose an aerobics shoe because it is more flexible.
weight training, stair climbing* and stationary biking	a cross trainer.
aerobics/dance exercise, weight training, stair climbing and biking	a cross trainer or aerobics shoe with a PU midsole.
aerobics/dance exercise and running	an aerobics shoe and a running shoe.
aerobics/dance exercise and fitness walking	an aerobics shoe and either a walking shoe or a running shoe.

*Step-training is included here.

for road and track running and with rubber tri-angles, squares, circles, or thick waves provide excellent *forward* movement, but since aerobic dance-exercise consists of forward, backward, and lateral movement, this is not the best choice of shoe sole.

"The rough treads of most running shoes can be hazardous during aerobic dance-exercise as they can cause the feet to come to an abrupt halt each time they strike the floor. Thus, most shoes designed for running are unsuitable for aerobic dance."[7]

▶ Do not select a wide heel flair of rubber if you have the tendency toward pronated ankles (lower leg bones do not sit directly on the ankle). This heel flair will not only limit, to some degree, your lateral (sideward) movement, but also it will not provide the appropriate correction to avoid future possible injury to naturally weak ankles, as it does in jogging — which is all forward movement. Pronation of ankles can best be corrected *inside* the shoe by means of:

▶ An *extra firm* heel box.

▶ Raising the arch with a specifically designed wedge.

▶ Controlling the floor contact of various portions of the foot by means of a specially designed orthotic (prescribed corrective device for the foot — Figures 5.1 and 5.2).

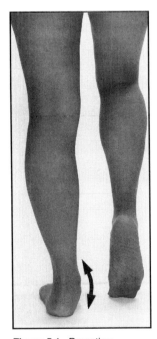 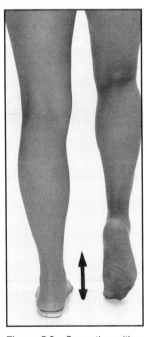

Figure 5.1. Pronation. **Figure 5.2.** Correction with a sports orthotic.

Structural Imbalances

The *sports orthotics* just mentioned are devices which are custom-made by hand to specifically control the function of your particular foot.

They are not arch supports. Requiring several weeks of construction, they are shaped to closely *control your foot the entire time it is on the ground.* The bones in your foot are now moved so that muscles can function and adapt normally, decreasing or eliminating foot problems. They are made of an unbreakable, reinforced material and are worn inside your athletic shoe.[8]

So don't just live with the pain that structural imbalances cause, like aching on the entire bottom of the foot from the forward movement of running, or shin splints from the lateral movement of aerobics. You should seek the advice of a qualified specialist like a podiatrist before wearing sports orthotics.

SELECT PROPER CLOTHING

Choosing what to wear for the environment in which you are exercising is quite important. Safety, comfort, and ease of movement are the keys for aerobics apparel. Dress in layers. A warm-up sweat-suit or jogging suit will assist in increasing the temperature of your arm and leg muscles during the warm-up portion of the hour. On very warm, or highly humid and warm days, this, of course, is unnecessary. Select cotton material over others since it absorbs perspiration better than other fabrics. When cotton clothing becomes damp, the surrounding air causes the moisture to evaporate, and this will cool your body.

During the routines, you want to be free to move in all directions and sweat freely, so wear as little as possible, especially when the temperature and relative humidity are high.

Long, loose slacks should be avoided, as they can catch under the feet. Tight-fitting garments should be avoided, as they restrict flexibility. The best advice for someone vigorously exercising is to keep clothing to a comfortable minimum. This allows unrestricted motion and facilitates loss of excessive body heat.[9]

Just be sure that you do not wear too much cloth-ing and get overheated. Persons very overweight or obese are especially prime targets for overheating because they have a thick layer of fat tissue between internal organs and the outside layer of skin. It works like insulation and keeps internal heat in. This means that the internal body systems may overheat and cause heat exhaustion or heat stroke. So don't try to "sweat" water pounds off by wearing lots of clothing or rubber-lined sweatsuits. Sweat and water loss are your cooling mechanisms and are not to be used as a measurement for weight loss because water is *not* fat!

You want to prevent friction, so wear cotton socks that absorb sweat and have no wrinkles. They help keep your feet free from blisters and to keep your feet drier.

Finally, it is against all physiological principles to wear a towel around the neck during exercise. The major artery from the heart to the brain is located in the neck area and needs to be able to be cooled by exposure of the skin surface in that area to air.

FLUID INTAKE

Being able to perform aerobics depends upon the replacement of your water losses. Water serves as the principle means of transporting heat (and substances) within the body. In warm environments (meaning within a room or a geographical location), it is the *only* means of dispersing body heat. This is accomplished by the evaporation of released perspiration on the surface of the skin. When the room air contacts the sweat, the skin surface is cooled, and the cooling is then internally conducted.

The production of body heat is greatly increased during physical exercise. *Unless water for perspiration is available, the body temperature increases beyond normal and there is overheating.* Thus, when fluid loss exceeds supply, dehydration follows, with an accompanying limited ability to exercise. When dehydration occurs, even modest physical activity causes the heart rate and body temperature to increase. When the water loss is approximately 5 percent of the total body water, evidence of heat exhaustion may become apparent, and when losses total 10 percent, the condition may soon lead to heat stroke, which is fatal unless cared for immediately (i.e., an ice bath submersion).

It is imperative that fluid intake be increased to maintain fluid balance as the work level and environmental temperature increase.[10]

Since there is no basis for restricting water intake during an aerobics hour and no evidence that humans can "adapt" or be "trained" to tolerate water intake that is lower than your daily losses, you should practice the habit of replacing water loss by continuous daily fluid intake.

A few guidelines to facilitate water balance are:

1 Drink plenty of liquids at least twenty minutes before the beginning of an aerobics hour. Frequent small intakes of fluid throughout the day is best.

2 For most sessions, if you have been providing plenty of water *prior* to the aerobics hour, you probably will not need to intake water *during* the hour (room temperature and humidity are the variables that usually determine this.) However, if you get thirsty during an hour, *do not hesitate to drink water.* Your thirst mechanism is even a *late* sign that you need water, so don't ignore it!

3 After an aerobics hour, relax and sit with a tall glass of ice water or inexpensive homemade electrolyte ("sports drink") solution, shown below. This will provide immediate rehydration and is a pleasant way to conclude your hour "to yourself."

"Homemade" electrolyte solution[11]

1 Qt. frozen reconstituted orange juice
3 Qts. water
1/2 Tsp. salt.

Deliberate dehydration (by loading on the clothes and promoting profuse sweating), of course, is not an acceptable method for weight control. This will cause a temporary loss of weight that is rapidly regained by rehydration. Loss of weight should only be body fat, *never* water or protein.

4 Many "sports beverages" are promoted as sources of available sodium, potassium and sugar. Replacement needs for sodium and potassium can be met much better by eating a diet that includes a variety of foods and supplies these and other nutrients — including proper amounts of water. If the athlete uses any of the "sports beverages" or commercial preparations, they should be diluted with water to decrease the concentration of sugar and thus decrease the time the fluid stays in the stomach. Recommended dilutions are given below.[12]

DILUTION FACTOR

The following replacement fluids should be diluted:

Fruit Juices	1 part juice; 3 parts water
Soft Drinks	1 part pop; 3 parts water
Vegetable Juices	1 part juice; 1 part water
Gatorade®	1 part drink; 1 part water
Pripps Pluss®	1 part drink; 3 parts water
Quickick® (orange flavor)	1 part drink; 3 parts water

But Remember — Water is the Best Replacement Fluid

COMMON INJURIES

Blisters

Blisters come in seconds and take days to heal. Even a small blister that goes uncared for will bother your workout. The best advice is to do everything you can to prevent them from forming.

Blisters are caused by friction as the surface of your shoe rubs against the skin of your foot. Make sure that your shoes fit well — not too loose and not too tight. To assist in the prevention of blisters, one simple procedure is to lubricate the trouble spot with petroleum jelly before you put your shoes on for another fitness session. If you sweat a lot, powder your feet also. Improper-fitting shoes are the culprit, so be sure that you do a few exertive moves in your local shoe store to size up comfort *in motion* before you purchase the shoes.

If you get a water blister, care for it as follows:

▶ Gently scrub the area with soap and water to thoroughly clean the area.

▶ Gently swab with alcohol or a surgical preparation.

▶ Make two incisions at the outer edges of the blister. Slowly press out the superficial fluid. Apply ointment or first-aid cream and bandage until healed completely.

If you get a blood blister, care for it as follows:

▶ Ice the area.

▶ Do not puncture. The chance of infection is great, since you are in immediate connection with your circulatory system.

▶ Place a "donut"-type compress around the blister until it is reabsorbed and completely healed.

Bunions

A bunion is a large bony protuberance on the outside of the big toe that indicates joint inflammation. The principle causes of bunions are overpronation and faulty foot structure. Seeking correction from a podiatrist is your plan of action.

Cramps (Muscle)

A cramp is a painful spasm of muscle. Cramping may occur during or following a vigorous exercise session and is the result of two different phenomena. Muscle cramping *during* an exercise session is primarily due to an electrolyte and fluid imbalance in your system.[13] Electrolytes are sodium, calcium, chloride, potassium, and magnesium. Cramping occurs primarily because you have not, with regularity, properly replaced your water intake as you condition and train.

If a great deal of sweating has occurred (eight or more pounds of water), replacement of those elements may be obtained by drinking, in solution (never in table form), a substance that replaces them. With moderate sweating and water loss, regular, daily water intake and proper diet will replace the needed fluids and electrolyte elements and do much to eliminate this type of cramping.

The most common cramps associated with exercise are those that occur in the *twenty-four hours after* exercise, especially after having gone to bed and/or after a sudden movement. These cramps (post-exercise) are not associated with electrolyte imbalance.[14] They are believed to be caused by muscle fiber swelling, causing then the agitation of (peripheral) nerves servicing the muscle tissue. If these cramps are frequent and severe, treatment is usually prescribed by taking .2 grams of quinine sulfate.

Immediate relief for either type of cramping is to *static stretch in the exact opposite direction* for a few moments.

Night Leg Cramps

Night leg cramps are usually caused by the position of the foot (bent down). Prescription: stretching exercises during the day and sleep positions which allow the foot to remain perpendicular to the leg.[15]

Side Stitch

A side stitch is the sharp pain in the side and usually represents a spasm of the diaphragm, the lower portion of the breathing mechanism. It is believed that side stitches occur primarily because not enough oxygen is getting to the area. This is due to a decreased blood flow to the location and most frequently occurs in those who have recently had a meal or drunk large volumes of fluid.

To help alleviate this phenomenon, immediately inhale deeply and bend forward from the waist, making the stomach and intestines push up against the diaphragm, using either a sitting (Figure 5.3) or standing position. Then, "tune in" to your breathing and consciously control your exhale. Do this by forming your lips as if you were going to whistle, and exhale through your puckered lips about five to ten times. For some, this seems to help.

The more conditioned person rarely experiences this type of pain, so prevention lies in continuing your program with regularity, with special attention to strength activities for the abdominal area.

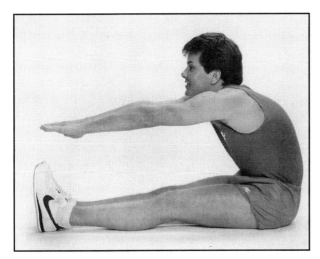

Figure 5.3. Side stitch relief.

Muscle Soreness

Two types of pain are associated with severe muscular exercise: (1) pain during and immediately after exercise, which may persist for several hours, and (2) a localized soreness that usually does not appear for twenty-four to forty-eight hours. The first is associated with the presence of metabolic wastes on pain receptors, the second with torn muscle fibers and/or connective tissue.[16] The immediate type need not be cause for great concern — it presents no lasting problems. The delayed type needs attention in the form of a more adequate warm-up and cool-down stretching program, and the incorporation of concluding strength activities. Gradual, sensible muscle use during exercise is the best prevention.

Muscle, Tendon, and Joint Injuries

1

For **muscle strains or sprains,** you **I.C.E.**: Ice, Compress, and Elevate. Injuries are iced (or cold whirlpools are administered) to inhibit swelling and promote healing by making the body internally (rather than at the surface) supply more blood to the affected deep-problem area. The body forces more blood to come to the area when cold applications are applied by making the body work harder pumping away the old cells and pumping in fresh oxygen and nutrients to begin the repair process at the deep site rather than at the surface skin area. Ice applications are administered two times a day for about twenty minutes. When the affected area no longer is warm to the touch (using the back of your hand), but seems to be the same temperature as the rest of the leg, arm, etc., ice compresses can be stopped.

When heat is applied, it brings an increase of blood to the skin surface, but it doesn't make the body work hard at all — on its own — to pump in a fresh supply of oxygen and nutrients to the *deep* affected area. So stick with the less comfortable ice measure, and your repair process will quicken.

2

Anchilles tendonitis is an inflammation of the thick tendon that connects the heel to the calf muscle. This injury is due to the use of shoes with inadequately thick heels, or which for some other reason do not provide a proper cushion for the foot. Biomechanical problems like the following aggravate the situation: bowed legs, tight hamstrings and calves, high-arched rigid feet, overpronation, and excessive toe-running.

To prevent Achilles tendonitis, perform adequate heel-cord stretching, and *don't exercise* with the pain. Aggravation of this problem can cause a serious and permanent condition.

Shin Splints

The most frequent injury experienced by new aerobics enthusiasts is shin splints. Shin splints is the term given to pain felt on the front and inside of the lower leg (Figure 5.4). Although a common affliction of runners, this malady can affect anyone who engages in physical activity which uses the legs. Most cases of shin splints occur in the *beginning* of an exercise program because the lower leg muscles are weak.

Jumping and running activities cause the leg muscles in the back of the leg to develop and become

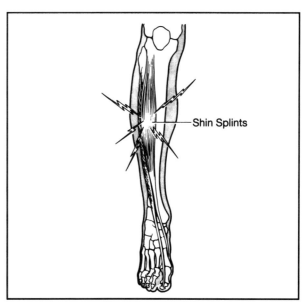

Figure 5.4. Shin splints.

stronger, while the leg muscles in front develop only slightly. This muscle imbalance can cause the disabling pain called "shin splints" if not treated correctly.[17]

When the strength of one muscle or muscle group is disproportionate to that of the antagonist(s) for that muscle or group, the weaker muscle should be strengthened to restore balance around the joint.[18]

Preventative measures are the first step with any exercise regimen. Light, flexible shoes with good arch support are mandatory. Stretching before and after physical activity also helps the muscles absorb shock. Avoid track running; the repeated turns put great stress on the lower leg.

Performing three repetitions of straight-leg and bent-knee wall leans for twenty seconds may help alleviate the problem (Figure 5.5).

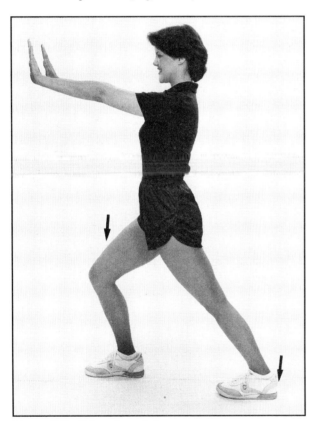

Figure 5.5. Shin splint relief.

Another preventative measure is to develop the strength of the anterior lower leg area. This can be accomplished by performing an exercise like the lower-leg flexor, which uses the resistance/rubber tubing. Sit tall with your legs together in front of you and place the center of the tubing under the toes of your shoes. Hands are comfortable in front of abdomen area and they don't move during the exercise. Slowly point your toes down & toward the wall

in front of you (Figure 5.6) and hold 15 seconds. Relax a few seconds and then flex your feet at the ankle, and draw your toes up tightly toward your knees (Figure 5.7) and hold 15 seconds. Repeat entire exercise for several minutes. This can be done one leg at a time or both feet working together, simultaneously.

Of utmost importance in the caring for shin splints are *rest and immediately icing* the area of tenderness. The icing should be done for eight to ten continuous minutes by means of gently massaging the problem area. Later in the day, a second gentle ice massage for the same duration of time should begin to give the desired relief. Continue this procedure for several days. You'll be amazed how quickly you "repair" within one week!

Also, you can minimize the discomfort by taking four to six aspirin a day. Toe raises on the edge of a step can help strengthen the posterior muscles which are heavily used in any running, jumping, or dancing

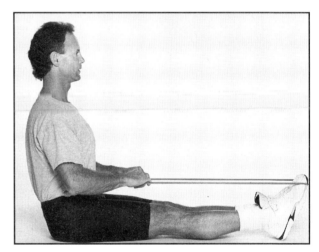

Figure 5.6. Strength exercise to develop the anterior lower leg muscles — **down** position.

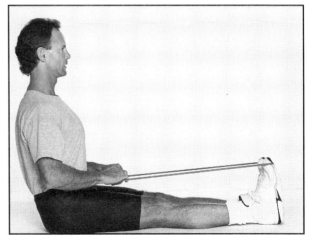

Figure 5.7. Strength exercise to develop the anterior lower leg muscles — **up** position.

activity. Walking on your heels with your toes in the air for thirty to sixty seconds is an easy way to build up strength in the front leg muscles. Pressing down on the heel of the fully extended leg while cycling also helps. Practice this stretch at traffic lights when you must wait.

If icing, rest, aspirin, strengthening, and stretching do not create relief within ten days, see a physician to rule out the more serious conditions such as stress fractures, structural imbalances which might require orthotics, or anterior compartment syndrome.[19]

DRUG USAGE AND POTENTIALLY FATAL EFFECTS ON THE HEART

It is believed that as many as half of all heart attack deaths occur because of "electrical failure" of the heart, not "pump failure." People with perfectly adequate amounts of heart muscle die because their heart's electrical signals go out of sync; the muscle then twitches chaotically and can no longer pump blood. Known as *ventricular fibrilation*, this rhythm disturbance is absolutely deadly if it cannot be reversed within minutes.[20] Drug-related deaths of superstar athletes (i.e., cocaine intoxication of recent years) is directly related to this phenomenon.

SEEK THE PROFESSIONALS

Understanding the cause and effect will help you to prevent problems or injuries during your quest for fitness. Whenever problems or injuries do occur, don't just "live with it." Seek out answers from the qualified professionals — medical doctors, sports medicine specialists and physiologists, or athletic trainers.

Within any body of information, misconceptions arise from unresearched statements promoted by individuals *not qualified* to make the statements. Many of the myths about the harm that exercise supposedly causes, or unscientific ideas concerning proper diet and exercise programs are being put to rest through better education.

For instance, several persons who are TV and movie personalities talk about "go for the burn." Key fitness research professionals have stated the opposite. "Don't try to achieve what some aerobic programs call the *burn*." A burning sensation in the chest could mean heart or coronary problems. If other muscles feel as if they were burning, it's probably a signal of overwork or injury approaching!"[21]

This text has been written to assist you, the novice, in understanding how your body works and how to improve it in various unique ways. Its design is purely *educational* in nature. It will provide you with a firm base so that *you* can evaluate the various programs and products being highly promoted these days in such areas as diet, exercise, mental training, etc.

The hope for your ongoing commitment to fitness is that you will refer to the most qualified sources available to answer your continual questions. People who are medical doctors (especially those who are "wellness" and "preventive medicine" oriented), physiologists and sports medicine specialists, i.e., the professionals who devote their entire working day and lives to researching and understanding human physiology — are overwhelmingly more qualified to advise you on a diet, exercise, or mental training program than a commercially oriented person. Glamorous movie and TV personalities sell you on their "expertise" by their media notoriety, their photogenic bodies and smiles, and the price tag attached to their information.

So be selective. Follow the diet, exercise, and mental training programs promoted by the *scientific professionals*. Choose to read and believe authors whose credentials are impressive in the various fields of total fitness and who publish their researched findings in *professional journals*. You will then have provided yourself with the most accurate, up-to-date knowledge available, and a more safe, fun way to good health.

Chapter 6

Posture: Good Positioning Underlies All Movement

Probably the key reason to include posture information in an aerobics course is to *save your back!* In order to insure that you are performing exercises in the *safest* possible fashion, you must understand good postural techniques, regardless of the activity you're performing. Developing good postural habits will insure that your spine is always held in a stabilized manner.

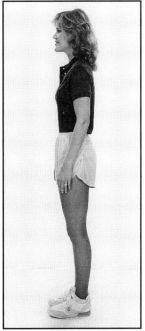 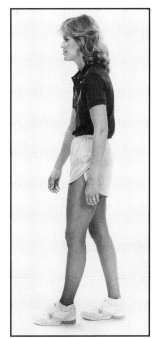

Figure 6.1.   **Figure 6.2.**

Posture is a choice!

UNDERSTANDING THE MECHANICS

The downward pressure of gravity applied to the bones of the upright, balanced skeleton will tend to cause it to buckle at three principal points: hip, knee, and ankle. And, since the weight of the body is largely in front of the spinal column, the body will tend to fall forward. To counteract these tendencies toward buckling and falling forward, we have five muscles, or muscle groups, which are designed to be "anti-gravity" in nature and which allow for an upright, balanced skeleton. Figure 6.3 shows these muscles and their relationship to the upright skeleton. These "anti-gravity" muscle groups that are responsible for holding us erect are located in the:

▶ Back, along the spinal column.

▶ Abdomen.

▶ Buttocks.

▶ Front of the thighs.

▶ Calves.

To develop good posture, the position of the spine, pelvic girdle, and hip joints (which act as the main hinges of the body) need to be controlled, and is done so primarily by the five muscle groups. *How* you control them determines a *good* posture.

CORRECT POSTURE AWARENESS

Safe, efficient positions for the performance of exercise and all daily living tasks are ones in which the various body segments are balanced — one above

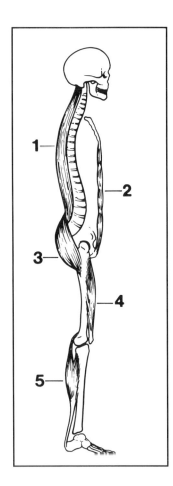

Figure 6.3.
Anti-gravity
muscle groups.

constantly having to work against it. Efficiency is thus obtained.

BALANCED POSTURES STATIC/DYNAMIC

A balanced standing posture is established by having:

▶ The head and *stretched* neck balanced on top of the spine and centered above the shoulders, keeping your chin parallel to the floor.

▶ Your shoulders pulled *back* and *down* (in a relaxed position).

▶ Your chest and rib cage raised *up*.

▶ Your abdominal muscles pulled *in and up*, under the rib cage.

▶ The pelvic girdle pulled *down and under*, tightening the buttocks. The pelvis rests on the two thigh bones balanced over two arched feet.

▶ Your knees *relaxed*. Locking your knees in a hyperextended position causes imbalance and makes you more susceptible to knee injury.

▶ Your weight distributed equally on both feet while standing with the feet *parallel* and toes pointing forward as you take the weight on the *outer* half of the feet.

▶ Your arms *relaxed*.

These key positions apply to standing. If each body segment is balanced, a vertical line should extend from the tip of the ear through the center of the shoulder, slightly behind the center of the hip, behind the kneecap, and just in front of the ankle joint. Whenever one part moves out of this line (as shown in Figure 6.4), your center of gravity shifts in the *direction* of that movement. Another part of you must then adjust in the opposite direction in order to maintain the center of gravity back over your base of support. Keeping this in mind will assist you in establishing the balancing, or "correct postural awareness," mentioned earlier to enable you to move well in any position and direction you choose — using stationary moves such as lunges and widestride varieties, or dynamic moves such as rocking, jogging, and bench-stepping.

POOR POSTURE: A HABIT THAT CAN BE CHANGED!

If any segment is out of body alignment, your weight distribution will be uneven over your base of

another. This ensures that a minimum of uneven pressure and friction occurs in the weight-bearing joints and that a minimum amount of strain occurs in the adjoining muscles, ligaments, and tendons. Initially in the learning process, you need to develop a kinesthetic awareness (sensation of position, movement, tension, etc., of parts of the body) so that you feel uncomfortable when moving through tasks incorrectly or inefficiently (i.e., while using poor posture). As you then develop continual good postural awareness, you will begin to move in well-aligned positions automatically!

This awareness will also provide you with a margin for safety in each joint, so that an unexpected force won't immediately push the joint beyond its normal limits and cause injury. And when your body is in proper alignment, it is in the best, most efficient position to resist the downward pull of gravity with the least amount of negative stress and effort. *A balanced posture makes full and efficient use of the force of gravity (by aligning all parts) so that the pull is directly downward through the supporting parts.* This allows the muscles to do minimal work in maintaining the body in an erect position. The ligaments and muscles surrounding each joint hold the part in place, cooperating with the pull of gravity instead of

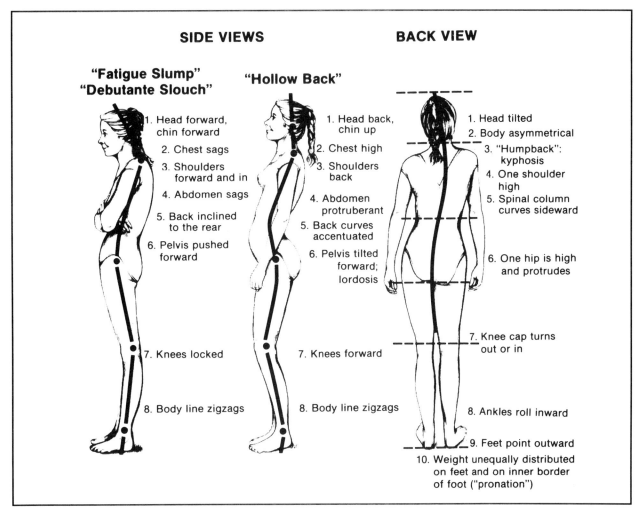

Figure 6.4. Poor Postures.

support and will put unnecessary strain on muscles, bones, and joints. This will soon cause fatigue.

Poor posture is very definitely a habit that can be changed, but it will take time — the habit that you now have has been a part of you for a long time. Because most muscles are in pairs, if a muscle is constantly shortened, its opposing muscle will lengthen and become weak from disuse. Therefore, stretching (lengthening) one set of muscles, while simultaneously contracting (shortening) the opposing set of muscles, *and then repeating vice versa,* will strengthen both (especially if additional weight resistance is used). With this thought in mind, you can understand why stretching and strengthening your muscles will develop an improved posture. For if your body is to move freely, every muscle needs to be able to shorten or lengthen in either a strong, quick manner or a slow, relaxed manner. Fully understanding the principles of both stretching and strength training will therefore assist you further in

understanding and obtaining your good posture goals.

EFFICIENT POSITIONS

If you now exhibit poor posture during aerobic movement activities, you will need to re-educate your neuromuscular system. This will take patience, persistence, and a sincere desire on your part to want to improve both your appearance and the efficiency of your body.

If you were born free from hereditary or congenital deformities, you *can* obtain good posture! It's all a matter of:

▶ Understanding balanced postures.

▶ Developing a kinesthetic awareness of your body positions during all movement.

▶ Developing strong, yet relaxed, muscles and flexible joints.

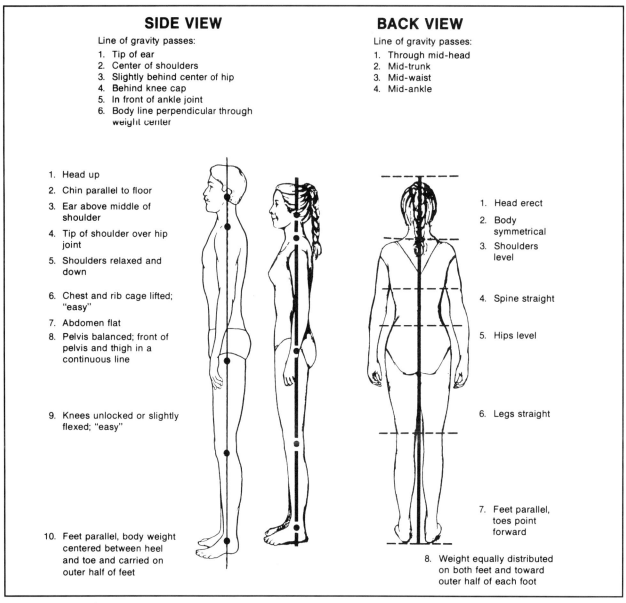

SIDE VIEW

Line of gravity passes:

1. Tip of ear
2. Center of shoulders
3. Slightly behind center of hip
4. Behind knee cap
5. In front of ankle joint
6. Body line perpendicular through weight center

1. Head up
2. Chin parallel to floor
3. Ear above middle of shoulder
4. Tip of shoulder over hip joint
5. Shoulders relaxed and down
6. Chest and rib cage lifted; "easy"
7. Abdomen flat
8. Pelvis balanced; front of pelvis and thigh in a continuous line
9. Knees unlocked or slightly flexed; "easy"
10. Feet parallel, body weight centered between heel and toe and carried on outer half of feet

BACK VIEW

Line of gravity passes:

1. Through mid-head
2. Mid-trunk
3. Mid-waist
4. Mid-ankle

1. Head erect
2. Body symmetrical
3. Shoulders level
4. Spine straight
5. Hips level
6. Legs straight
7. Feet parallel, toes point forward
8. Weight equally distributed on both feet and toward outer half of each foot

Figure 6.5. Good Postures.

▶ Desiring to obtain good posture.

▶ Discipline to continue what you have learned.

As you understand correct technique, challenge yourself to try using these positions for every total fitness component of your program, i.e., stretching, aerobics, and strength training exercises.

At first you'll be "thinking through" the activity, but with persistent practice and desire, you can exchange any former faulty habits for safe, more complimentary ones.

Stationary Purposes: If you can exhibit the balanced standing posture described and pictured earlier for activities that require a *stationary*, poised, controlled look, you've mastered this area already!

Dynamic Purposes: Performing the aerobic gesture and step patterns will require you to exhibit a different body position, or posture, than when you are just standing stationary and poised. These are the times when you are *preparing to move dynamically — in some direction through space* (forward, backward, laterally, up, down, etc.). While preparing to move through space, the broader your base of support, the lower your center of gravity (weight center) becomes. This, then, allows for better balance so that you can move quickly and more efficiently in any direction.

CORRECT LIFTING AND LOWERING

To protect your muscles and joints (especially the lower back) from undue strain or fatigue, proper efficient technique in these areas *must* become second nature to you. Disciplined practice of correct techniques *now* will establish good habits for the rest of your life. The leg muscles are very strong, whereas the back muscles are relatively weak. All heavy lifting should be done by stabilizing the back in an erect position and making the legs provide the necessary power.

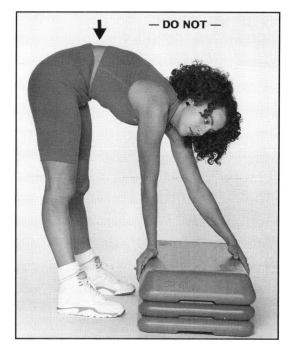

Figure 6.7.

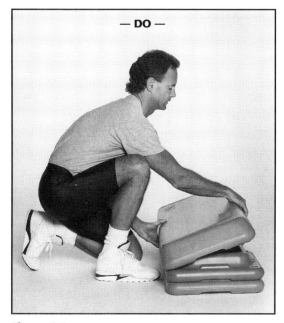

Figure 6.6.

1 Get as close to the object as possible, using a forward-stride position. The object should be in front of you if you are using two hands (i.e., step-bench) or beside you if you are using one hand (i.e., luggage). Keep your back straight and your pelvis tucked, and bend at the hips, knees, and ankles to lower your body. Lower directly downward, only as much as necessary.

2 Both arms should be placed well under and/or *around the weight center* of the load. Lift vertically upward in a slow, steady movement by extending your leg muscles. Keep the object close to your weight center. (Figure 6.6). Reverse the procedure to lower the object.

Do not:

Bend over from the hips (head low, buttocks high) and allow your back muscles to lift the load (Figure 6.7).

CORRECT CARRYING

1 Keep the object close to your weight center.

2 Separate the load when feasible, and carry half in each hand/arm.

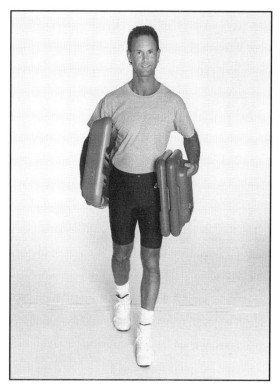

Figure 6.8.

DEVELOPING YOUR POSTURAL AWARENESS THROUGH POSTURE EXERCISES

Exercising the anti-gravity muscles is a fundamental part of any total physical fitness conditioning program. In order to develop and then maintain a good posture, these muscles need to be:

▶ **Strong** enough to perform their functions.

▶ **Flexible** enough to allow a variety of movement.

▶ **Relaxed** enough to perform with ease.

Therefore, establishing a program of strength exercises for the abdomen, lower back, hip, thigh, and calf areas will help you to obtain a balanced pelvic alignment and provide the means for efficient and painless movement. And, as mentioned, each joint involved needs to be flexible enough to permit the full range of movement possible from these groups of anti-gravity muscles so that any new position can be properly maintained. The three exercises in this chapter will help you to develop joint flexibility of the anti-gravity muscle groups needed to maintain correct postures. And establishing a program of relaxation will assist with ease of performance, while moving or while motionless.

However, the *best* exercise that you can do for yourself is both a physical and mental one: *Become aware of correct postural technique with every move you make.* Then practice this physical and mental conditioning constantly until it becomes a habit — until it becomes you.

Note

Review the eight key cues for establishing good posture (i.e., chest up, shoulders down, etc.) and then proceed with the following exercises.

Elbows Wide 'N Close

To understand the awareness of "space between shoulder blades" *contracted* and then *widely stretched*, keeping chest raised in either direction:

Note

DO NOT tightly lace fingers BEHIND THE NECK. Pulling on the cervical spine is not a good body position technique.

1 Clasp your hands loosely behind your head (Figure 6.9). Keep your **elbows out and high**, shoulders down and chin parallel to the floor. **4 counts.**

2 Exhale, and widen the space between your shoulder blades by bringing elbows **together** in front of your nose (Figure 6.10). **Hold. 4 counts.**

3 Inhale, and return **elbows wide** to the sides (Figure 6.9). **4 counts.**

4 Exhale and pull your elbows **up and back**, tightly contracting the space between your shoulder blades. Hold. **4 counts**

5 Inhale and return **elbows wide** to the sides (Figure 6.9). **4 counts.**

6 For variety, repeat attempting to touch elbows together, first **in front of forehead** and **below the chin**, maintaining the good posture position.

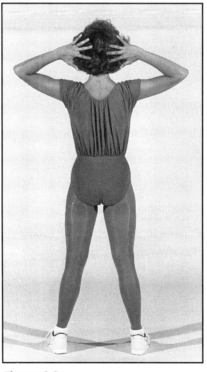
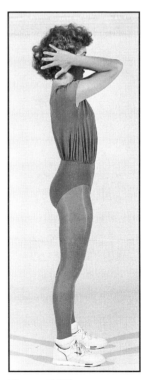

Figure 6.9.   **Figure 6.10.**

Cues

Elbows out and high, together, wide, up and back, wide.

Rib Lifter

To establish the awareness to the all-important position of "chest high" (and not sagging), this exercise will help to isolate and stretch the intercostal (rib) muscles:

1 **Stand** in correct alignment, with your **arms forward** and **parallel** to the ground. Place your thumbs and index fingers of each hand together, hands forward, palms down (Figure 6.11). **4 counts.**

2 Bend your elbows, bring your arms back, and place your palms parallel to the ground above your breast, with your **thumbs** snugly **under the armpits** and elbows held wide and parallel to the ground (Figure 6.12). **4 counts.**

3 Without lifting your shoulders or bending forward, **lift your entire rib section as high as you can**. Breathe deeply, inhale and exhale. 8 counts.

4 Now **lift** your elbow high **and stretch** rib cage on one side (Figure 6.13). **4 counts.**

5 **Lower** raised elbow to shoulder level. **4 counts.**

6 Repeat with lifting and lowering of other elbow. **8 counts.**

7 Repeat **raising both** together (Figure 6.14); **lower. 8 counts**

Cues

Stand; thumbs under armpits; lift ribs and breathe; lift and stretch, lower; repeat other side; repeat both.

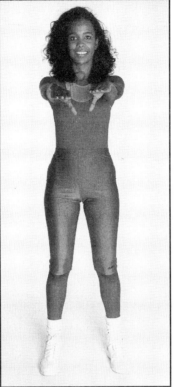

Figure 6.11.

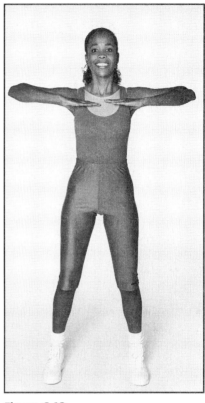

Figure 6.12.

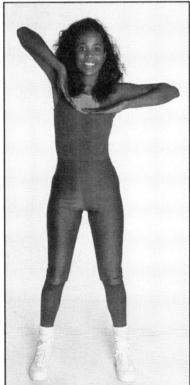

Figure 6.13.

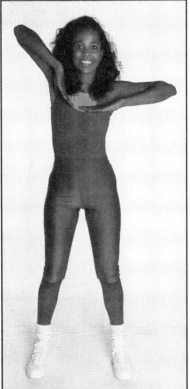

Figure 6.14.

Reaching Correctly

To establish the awareness in keeping the **shoulders back and down** as you perform arm movement that is forward and upward:

1 **Stand** in correct alignment. Place the back of your left hand on your central lower back and pelvic girdle area (Figure 6.15). **4 counts.**

2 Slowly **raise** your right arm forward and in front of your body above your head, keeping your lower arm and hand stationary, your elbow still flexed (Figure 6.16). **4 counts.**

3 Slowly **lower** your arm to its original position in standing alignment. **4 counts.**

4 Place the back of your right hand on your central lower back, and slowly **raise and lower** your left arm as before. **8 counts.**

5 With both arms lowered and both hands resting lightly on thighs, slowly **raise both arms** in front of your body and above your head in the same manner in which each was raised (Figure 6.17). **4 counts.**

6 Slowly **lower** to original position. **4 counts.**

7 Repeat all, once again. **24 counts.**

Cues

Stand; raise one and lower; raise opposite and lower; raise both and lower.

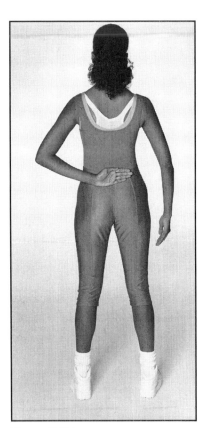

Figure 6.15.

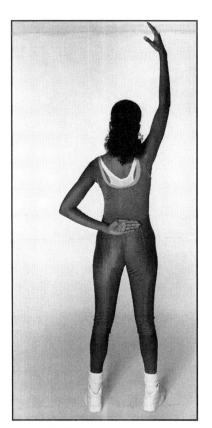

Figure 6.16.

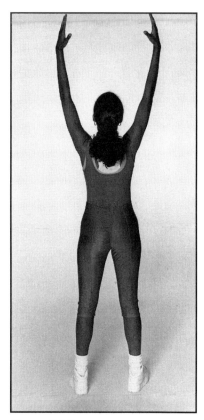

Figure 6.17.

POSTURE SUMMARY

For your total daily well-being, the development, continued awareness, and usage of good posture must become important enough to you to be a life-long endeavor. So start now! Are you sitting correctly while reading how to improve your posture? Think good posture at all times!

The knowledge of a well-aligned body and the development of a kinesthetic awareness (feeling) of good posture are the first steps toward acquiring good postural habits. This constant awareness of good posture —

▶ standing tall

▶ with chin parallel to the floor

▶ shoulders lowered and pulled back tight

▶ chest raised up

▶ pulling your abdomen first in and then up

▶ tucking your pelvis under

▶ and thereby making your torso erect

— is the one best exercise that you can physically and mentally do for yourself. *Then remember, too, when you are engaged in any exercise program, that to move efficiently and safely depends upon proper body alignment at all times and in all positions.*

Practicing on a daily basis is required for this to become an integral part of you. Good posture is only established through *discipline*. Setting aside time to perform techniques and exercises to encourage good posture and develop strength and flexibility, accompanied by constant attention to posture throughout your daily living tasks, will make this all become a reality to you. You can improve as you move—all day, every day—for this is where your total program for a fit physique begins!

Chapter

Program Techniques — Start to Finish

Complete background information needed to safely and efficiently enjoy an aerobics exercise program has been established in detail in the first six chapters. The rest of the text gives additional, ancillary information for each of the dimensions of a total physical fitness program.

The following chapter of aerobic techniques represents a visual resource of exercise movement depicting basic steps and gestures for each of the four key program segments (i.e., the warm-up, aerobic exercise/step training, strength training, and cool-down/flexibility training/relaxation). It also covers the unique portions of each of these segments. Brief directions accompany the techniques and they are photographed and described by the "mirroring technique." Therefore, follow the words and perform the movement exactly as shown.

I. THE WARM-UP SEGMENT

Note: The Warm-Up Segment includes active, low-level, rhythmic, limbering, standing, range-of-motion type of exercises for approximately five minutes, followed by five minutes of slow, sustained, static stretching from head to toe. Principles for each are described and shown in Chapter 4, Figures 4.1–4.4. With this information in mind, proceed with the following techniques.

▶ ACTIVE, LOW-LEVEL, RHYTHMIC, LIMBERING, STANDING MOVES

Figures 7.1–7.2.

Step-Touch

With big arm curl swings.
2 counts

(See 4.1 with arm circles.)

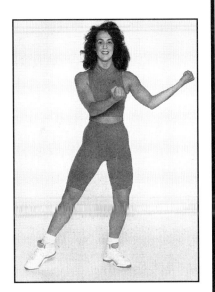

Figure 7.1.

Step-Out Wide and Squat

Hold, side-clap, side-clap.
4 counts

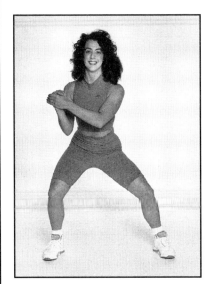

Figure 7.2.

▶ STATIC STRETCHING MOVES[1]

Figures [4.2–4.4; 4.20–4.22] 7.3–7.10

Shoulder Circles

Up, back, down, forward; or alternate, one at a time.
4 counts in each direction

(See 4.2 for Neck Stretch.)

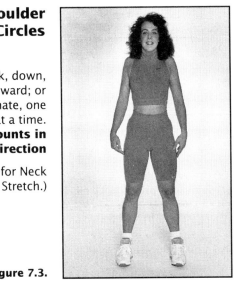

Figure 7.3.

Arm Sweeps

Low and center; wide and palms up; raise, reach high.
8 counts

Reverse
8 counts

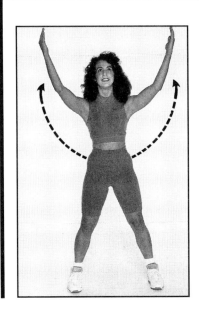

Figure 7.4.

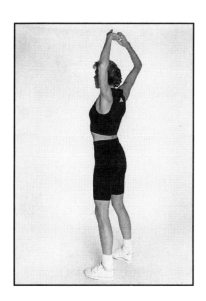

Chest

Grasp hands very high, elbows bent, press back, and hold.
8 counts

Figure 7.5

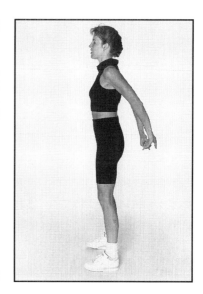

Chest

Grasp hands low, behind back, lift and hold.
8 counts

Figure 7.6

Low Back

Feet apart, hands on thighs; flatten back, hold.
8 counts

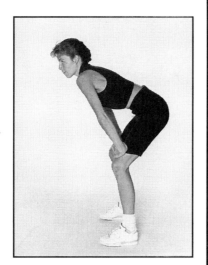

Figure 7.7.

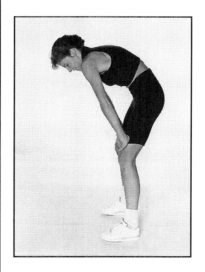

Low Back

Now round lower back upward, contract abdominals, tuck buttocks under hips, and hold.
8 counts

Figure 7.8.

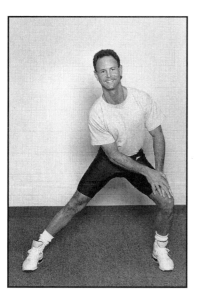

Inner Thigh

Feet apart/toes forward, shift weight/hips R, flex R knee over R toe, and hold.
8/16 counts

Reverse.

Figure 7.9.

Hip Flexors

Forward/back stride, feet forward, fists at waist; firmly tuck buttocks under hips, flexing knees/lowering elbows, and hold.
8/16 counts

Reverse.

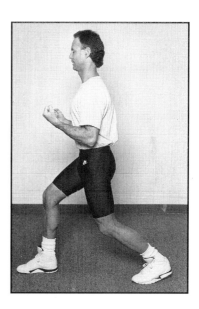

Figure 7.10.

II. THE AEROBIC SEGMENT

Note

Remember, any activity that promotes the supply and use of oxygen using the criteria established in Chapter 2 can be performed during this 20–60 minute segment of time. This includes the pace-walking and jumping rope detailed earlier, and the aerobics and bench-step training presented here.

Aerobics   Figures [4.5–4.19], 7.11–7.50

▶ LOW-IMPACT AEROBICS   Figures 7.11–7.28.

Bounce, Two Feet

Lift to the balls of both feet (parallel or forward/back stride) and lower.
1 quick count; or 2 counts

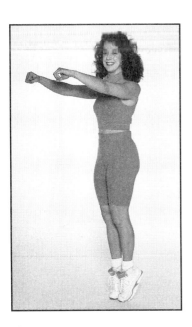

Figure 7.11.

Bounce 'n Hitch-Kick

One-foot bounce while bending other knee, with lower leg pointing back.
1 count

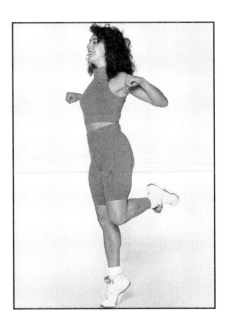

Figure 7.12.

One-foot bounce and kick same leg forward, waist-high or lower.
1 count

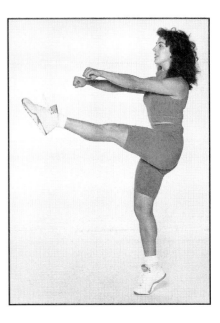

Figure 7.13.

▶ LOW-IMPACT AEROBICS

Bounce 'n Tap Series

One-foot bounce on L foot, pointing and tapping R toe forward. Arms punch parallel forward.
1–4 counts

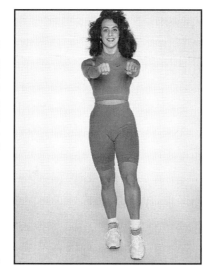

Figure 7.14.

Weight remains on L bouncing, R toe now pointing and tapping wide R. Arms follow, wide to sides, palms/fists up.
1–4 counts

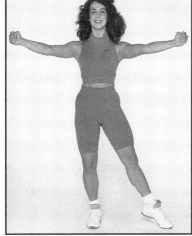

Figure 7.15.

Weight remains on L bouncing, R toe now pointing and tapping backward. Arms raise overhead, thumbs back.
1–4 counts

Next: Alternate by bringing pointing and tapping foot in, and two-foot bounce in place.
1–4 counts

Shift weight to R foot and repeat series.

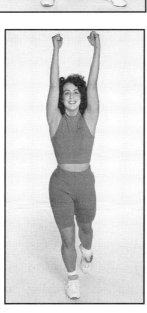

Figure 7.16.

Hoe-down

Bounce R foot, lifting L knee to L side. Arms parallel punch down.
1–2 counts

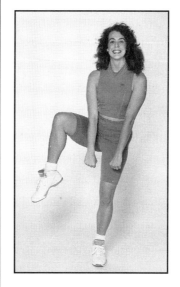

Figure 7.17.

Feet together bouncing. Arms lift chest-high in a half upright-row position. (Transitional move.)
1 count

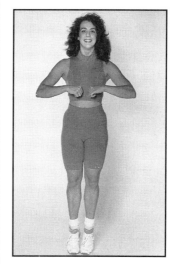

Figure 7.18.

Bounce L foot, extending R heel forward. Arms parallel punch down.
1–2 counts

Last, repeat Figure 7.18 transitional move.
1 count

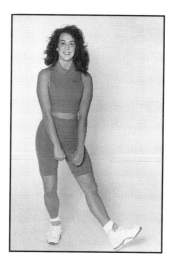

Figure 7.19.

▶ LOW-IMPACT AEROBICS

Heel-Toe Bounce Series

Bounce R foot
while L heel
extends forward.
Arms forward.
1 count

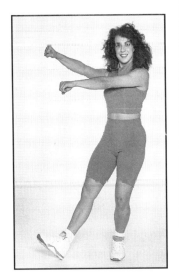

Figure 7.20.

Bounce R foot, while L
toe now taps in close.
Draw arms in to
chest.
1 count

Repeat heel out,
followed by feet back
in together in a
transitional move.
1 count

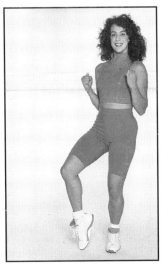

Figure 7.21.

Kicks

Weight on one
foot, kick other
leg to only a **90°
waist-high level**
(or lower).
Forward or
sideward.
1 count

Bounce added.
2 counts

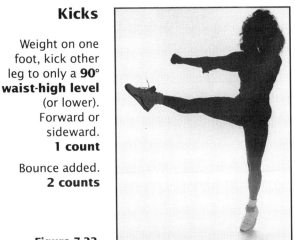

Figure 7.22.

Knee-Lift Varieties

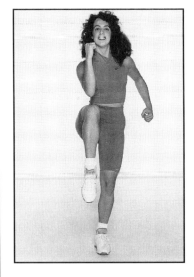

Step R, knee-lift
L knee forward,
same elbow touch.
2 counts

Reverse.

Figure 7.23.

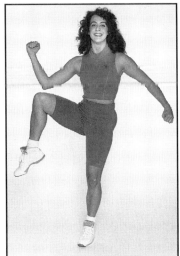

Step R, knee-lift
L knee sideward,
same elbow out-
wide and touch.
2 counts

Reverse.

Figure 7.24.

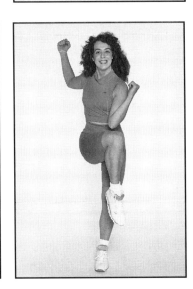

Step R, knee-lift
L knee across body
center forward,
R (i.e., opposite)
elbow across chest
and touching the
knee-lifted.
2 counts

Reverse.

Figure 7.25.

▶ LOW-IMPACT AEROBICS

Lunge Side and Bounce

Step and bounce-lunge R,
arms overhead, parallel, and
diagonally high L, head
following direction of arms.
2 counts

Reverse, shifting weight.
2 counts

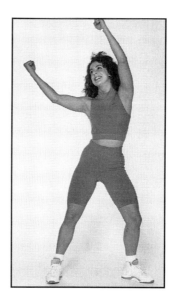

Figure 7.26.

Marching

Step-lift, one count
each step pattern.
Arms swing
opposite and **big.**
1 count

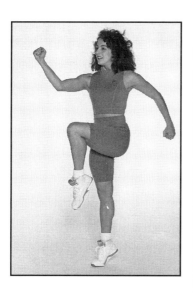

Figure 7.27.

Side Step-Out

Step out wide
stride to R side,
bending knees.
1 count

Clap hands R.
1 count

Reverse.
2 counts

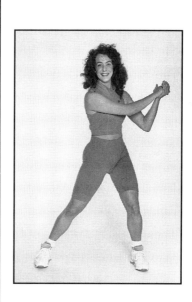

Figure 7.28.

Note

Remember, Low-Impact Aerobics are any exercise-dance movements in which one
foot always has contact with the ground and that fulfill the other aerobic criteria
established in Chapter 2.

▶ POWER LOW-IMPACT WITH PLYOMETRIC MOVES

Figures [2.13; 4.10–4.14] 7.29–7.32[2]

Two-Foot Jump

Step 1

Lift high on balls of feet, without leaving floor.
1 count

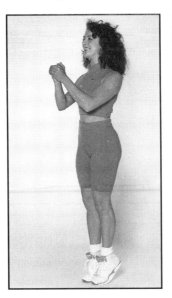

Figure 7.29.

Step 2

Land and gently **press the heels** into the floor.
1 count

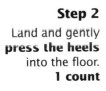
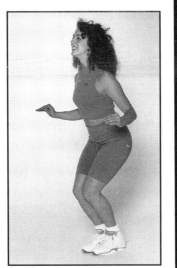

Figure 7.30.

Knee Lift

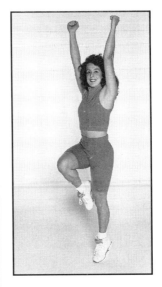

Lift knee while rising to **ball** of foot.
1 count

Be sure to lower heel of support foot, as lifted foot returns to ground.
1 count

Arms forcefully assist in **raising** entire body, reaching above shoulder level.

Figure 7.31.

Twist

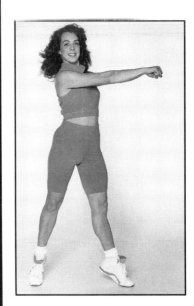

Shift weight from ball of foot, to ball of foot, as you lift your body and twist from side to side.
2 counts

Figure 7.32.

Note

You can easily use these moves as moderate impact plyometric moves—lunges [Figure 2.10-2.12], jumps, kicks, step-touches, jogs, heel-jacks, ponies.[3]

▶ HIGH-IMPACT AEROBICS

Figures [2.5 and 2.9; 4.15–4.16] 7.33–7.46

With high-impact locomotor (movements that take you from place to place through space) activities, you are briefly airborne and have **a take off** and **a landing**. The five basic high-impact locomotor movements are the following:[4]

Take-Off	Landing	Example	Figure
One foot	same foot	hop; hitch-kick	7.33; 7.34-7.35
One foot	opposite foot	leap; rock	7.36; 7.37-7.39
One foot	two feet	astride	7.40
Two feet	two feet	jump (together or wide-stride)	7.41-7.42
Two feet	one foot	hopscotch	7.43-7.44

The following are brief examples of the five basic take-offs and landings found in high-impact aerobics. Limit the repetitions of the same impact landing to **four or less**, so overuse and injury are avoided.

Hops — Single and Double

Hop R, forward lifting L knee.
1 count

For **Double Hops:**
Repeat R hop.
2 counts.

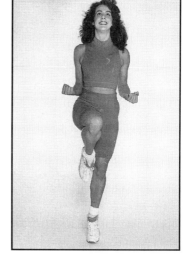

Figure 7.35.

Hitch-Kick

Step 1

Hop on L as R foot lifts back, knee bent.
Option:
Arms forcefully pulling back).
1 count

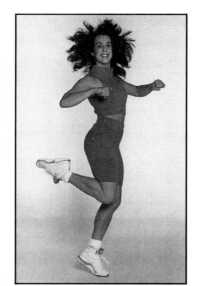

Figure 7.33.

Step 2

Hop L again, kicking R forward, waist-high or lower.
Option:
Arms forcefully parallel punching forward.
1 count

Reverse.
2 counts

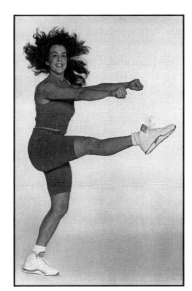

Figure 7.34.

Leap

With weight L (not shown) take-off, propelling body forward and upward, landing on R foot.
4 counts

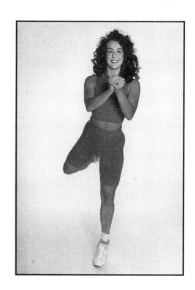

Figure 7.36.

Rock Side-To-Side

Hop on R foot to R side, placing weight over R leg (knee and ankle flexed), lifting L leg out to the side.
1 count

Reverse.

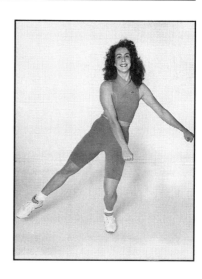

Figure 7.37.

▶ HIGH-IMPACT AEROBICS

Rock:

Forward

Rock (hop) R into a forward lean, lifting L leg back and up for balance.
1 count

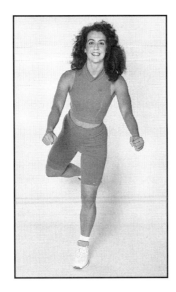

Figure 7.38.

Backward

Rock (hop) L backward into a backward lean, lifting R leg forward and up for balance.
1 count

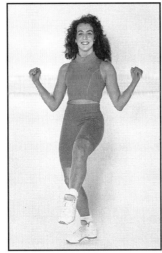

Figure 7.39.

Stride

Weight R or L (not shown) hop to astride or straddle position, loading weight onto both feet by bending knees.
1 count

(Usually preceded or followed with another move.)

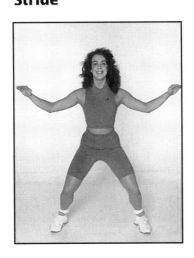

Figure 7.40.

Jumps:

Feet Together

Jump sideward, forward, or back. Hold.
2 counts
Reverse.
Option:
Use skiing arms position with L elbow **close**, R elbow high and wide, when jumping R. Reverse arms when you reverse feet.)

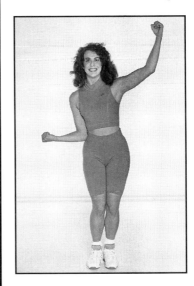

Figure 7.41.

Lunge or Wide-Stride

Two-foot scissors jump forward on R foot, bending R knee as L leg is kept extended back (still bearing weight on L) in wide forward/ backward lunge position. L arm forward, R arm back.
1 count

Options: Jump back to **two-feet together** and center, **1 count**, then reverse the forward and backward legs and arms lunging and jumping back to center.
2 counts.

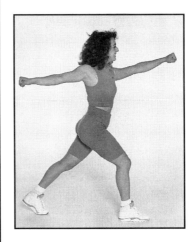

Or, reverse **directly** from forward/back-ward lunge, (1 count) to opposite forward/back-ward lunge position.
1 count

Figure 7.42.

Note

When executing two-foot jump to the side in wide-stride position, followed by two-foot jump together, this becomes a Jumping Jack (see 4.15–4.16). Arms can work wide and together with legs, or in opposition.

▶ HIGH-IMPACT AEROBICS

Hopscotch

Back

Hop to stride position (not shown), and with weight on L foot, hop and touch R foot raised **backward** to lowered L hand. **2 counts.** For balance, reach R hand diagonally skyward, thumb **back.** Reverse.

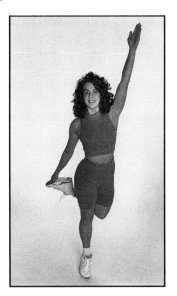

Figure 7.43.

Forward

Hop to stride position (not shown) and with weight on R foot, hop and touch L foot raised forward to lowered R hand (a knee open position). **2 counts.**

For balance, reach L hand diagonally skyward, thumb **back.** Reverse.

Note: If you have sensitive (injury-prone or recent surgery) knees, avoid this exercise variety.

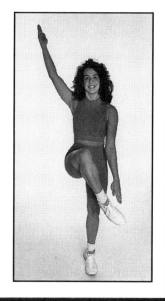

Figure 7.44.

Note

Many established popular social dances, or dance steps and gestures, are incorporated in the aerobics class setting.[5]

Polka

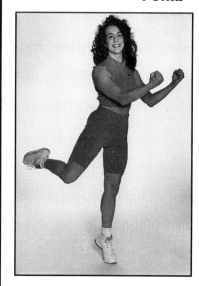

Step 1

Hop R, lifting L leg backward.

1 count

Figure 7.45.

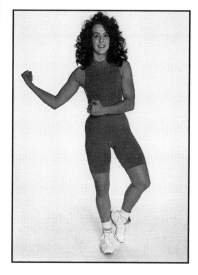

Steps 2–4

Step L, in close quickly.

½ count

Step R, in close quickly.

½ count

Step L, in close quickly.

½ count

Figure 7.46.

▶ HIGH / LOW-IMPACT AEROBICS   Figures [4.15–4.17]

This section of the aerobics class setting was described in depth in Chapters 2 and 4, so techniques can be reviewed there. Most **high-impact** moves can be easily converted to **low-impact** moves simply by removing the five basic high-impact locomotor movements just detailed. Instead of a take-off and landing, those moves are changed to moves:

▶ incorporating one foot remaining on the ground, as the fre foot uses floor and air space; or

▶ keeping both feet on the ground, incorporating the lifting and lowering plyometric principles in Chapter 2.

And, to change the low-impact moves to high-impact, you simply replace the stationary-foot move, and incorporate the high-impact locomotor moves of take-offs and landings (i.e., hops, hitch-kicks, leaps, rocks, hop astride, two-foot jumps, or hopscotch-type moves replace a low-impact "step" move).

▶ AEROBICS VARIETY: FUNK MOVES!   Figures 7.47-7.50

Funk aerobics are exercise moves developed from the culturally rich areas of jazz dance, ballet, street dance, gymnastics floor-exercise competition, and other rhythmical forms of aesthetic, emotionally expressive movement.

Funk aerobics include numerous expressive trunk, elbow and knee moves (Figure 7.47), funk walking (Figure 4.48) mimicking movie and television characters, and animation moves like "doing the Roger Rabbit" or funky chicken.

Creative expression and attitude prevail in funk exercise movement. Body gestures include the extremely big and wide-open positions (Figure 7.49), followed quickly with closed, tight, head gesture or hair-tossing moves (Figure 7.50).

You'll find the only limitations for funk aerobics movement lies in your own resources of experience and your individual creativity — which for all of us is absolutely unlimited!

Elbows and Knees

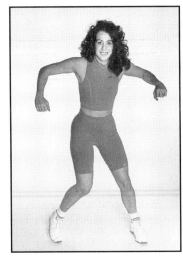

Figure 7.47.

Walks and Animation

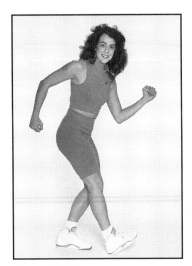

Figure 7.48.

Open

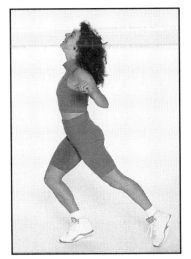

Figure 7.49.

Closed

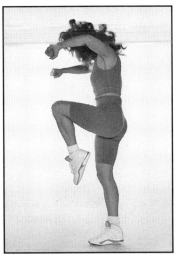

Figure 7.50.

Summary of Aerobics Techniques

Low-Impact, Power Low-Impact, Moderate Impact, High-Impact, and "Combo" have been described and detailed here so that you can design an individualized program according to your needs. Chart 15 in the Appendix is provided for you to develop an individualized program, incorporating your favorite impact moves, in combinations you choose. Chapter 8 (Choreography) will assist you in designing a safe, challenging, and fun aerobics program.

Remember, the aerobic segment of your program can include many varieties: pace walking/jogging/running, jumping rope, cycling, swimming, cross-country skiing, etc., and the newest aerobics exercise modality that is taking the fitness industry by storm — step training and the use of light resistance while stepping.

BENCH/STEP TRAINING

Figures [4.45–4.50], 7.51–7.96

Note

Techniques introducing the bench/step training with regard to bench height to choose, proper technique for stepping up and stepping down, and adding hand-held weights to increase intensity and further promote upper-body conditioning are described and shown in Chapter 4, Figures 4.45–4.50.

How you initially approach (step your first step of a pattern onto the bench), correct step-training posture to avoid injuries, the basic step movements, and how to add variety to the basic step movements and patterns is all presented here. Encouraging you to create your own individual step movements and pattern combinations concludes this section with Chart 15 in the Appendix entitled "Creating Your Own Step-Training Pattern Variations and Aerobic Exercise Routines."

▶ BENCH/STEP DIRECTION APPROACHES

Figures 7.51–7.55

Note

If you're following the movements of an instructor, position the bench for maximum visibility. Initial movement onto the bench can begin from one of the five following directions — the direction in which your body faces the bench.

From the Front

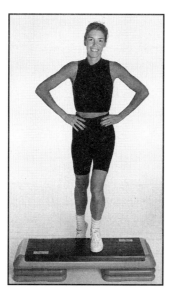

Facing the bench squarely.

Figure 7.51.

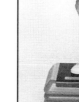

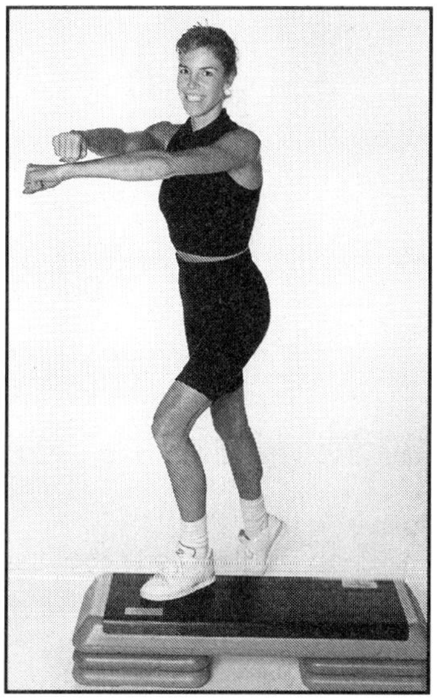

Facing on an angle toward corner when beginning a by-pass pattern (i.e., second move "by-passes" the bench and is a knee-lift, kick, etc.).

Figure 7.52.

From the Side

Standing with **your side** next to the bench's **side**, step up with foot that is closest to the side of the bench.

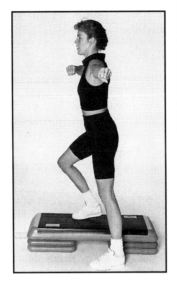

Figure 7.53.

From the Top

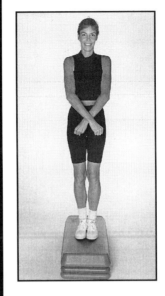

Atop, facing the bench's **end**, with feet together (shown); or feet in a forward/backward stride.

Figure 7.55.

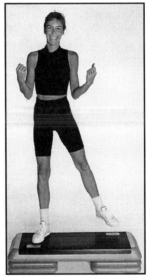

Atop, facing bench's **front**, with feet apart (shown); or feet together.

Figure 7.56.

From the End

Facing the **end** of the bench, step up and down.

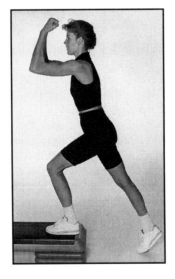

Figure 7.54.

Astride/ Straddle

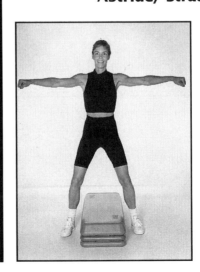

Facing the bench's **end**, standing astride or straddle position, with bench between your feet.

Figure 7.57.

▶ CORRECT STEP-TRAINING POSTURE

Figures 7.58–7.63

Here are three common step-training errors to avoid. The man is demonstrating incorrect postural techniques for each exercise, and the woman is performing correctly. Additional performance suggestions are also given.[6]

These moves are important to include for muscle balance

(1) **Hip/Leg Extension**

Some participants create an undesirable curve of the lower back with an excessive rear leg lift and exaggerate the problem with a forward body lean.

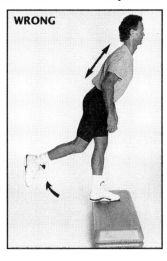
Figure 7.58.

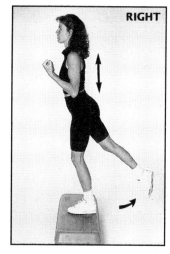
Figure 7.59.

Stand tall on the platform and extend the rear lifting leg **back** not up.

These moves are great exercises for the thighs and buttocks

(2) **Side Step-Out Squats**

Some participants have a tendency to lean too far out to the side, which places too much stress on the knee.

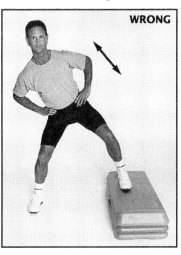
Figure 7.60.

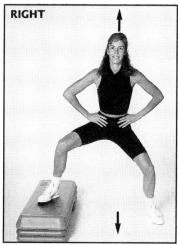
Figure 7.61.

Balance your weight evenly, keeping your center of gravity squarely within your legs.

(3) **Step-Back Lunges From Platform**

Do not bend too far forward at the hip or have your leg reaching back in a locked-knee position. Also, heel should not be forced to the ground; this position may be too much dorsiflexion of the foot for you.

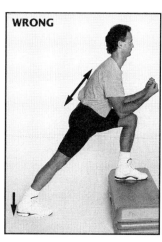
Figure 7.62.

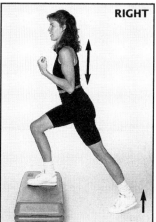
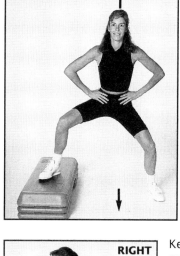
Figure 7.63.

Keep your body weight predominantly over the platform leg and keep your knee over your toes. The leg reaching back should make floor contact, with your knee slightly flexed. This will help reduce any chance of joint trauma from ground impact. Back heel is raised up off the floor.

▶ STEP-TRAINING BASIC STEP PATTERNS[7]   Figures 7.64–7.76

Note

Basic steps are organized here by the direction you initially approach the bench. They are identified as a:

▶ "**single** lead step" in which the **same** foot leads **every four count cycle**; or as

▶ an "**alternate** lead step" — the right and left foot both serve as the lead foot **alternately initiating every 4 counts** requiring a complete cycle for the alternating patterns to **take 8 counts** (i.e., both the right foot and then left foot lead a 4-count portion of the cycle).

For both safety and variety, when using single-lead-step, 4-count cycle patterns, lead with the right foot for a **maximum of one minute**, and then change to a left-foot lead. To accomplish this change in lead foot (for single cycle 4-count step patterns), perform a **non-weight-bearing, transitional, hold/touch/tap/heel** move as the last step of the cycle, initiating the change, with that foot. Within the descriptions, only the moves typed in bold face are shown in the Figures.

▶ BENCH APPROACH — FROM THE FRONT

Basic Bench Step

Single lead step, **4 counts.**

	R	L	R	L	
Right Lead:	**up**	up	down	**down**	4 counts

	L	R	L	R	
Left Lead:	up	up	down	down	4 counts

Arms shown: Long-lever punching on up, up; pull, punch, on the down, down.

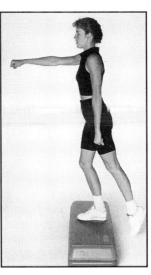 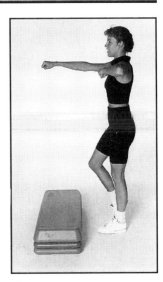

Figure 7.64.   **Figure 7.65.**

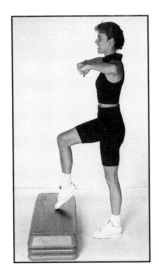

Step Tap

Single lead step, **4 counts.**

```
        R   R
```
Bench-tap down; repeat with left foot.
4 counts

Arms shown: Elbows shoulder-high, fists together on tap; fists apart on down.

Figure 7.66.

▶ STEP-TRAINING BASIC STEP PATTERNS

Single Cycle Bench-Tap

Alternating lead step.
8 counts.

R   L   L   R
Up **bench-tap** down down

Alternate (i.e. Up (L), bench-tap (R), down (R), down (L).

Arms shown:
Forward punching.

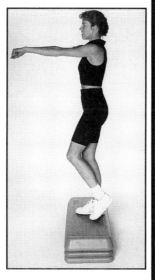

Figure 7.67.

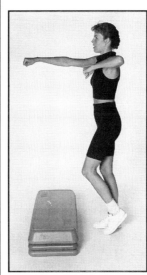

Single Cycle Floor-Tap

Alternating lead step,
8 counts.

R   L   R   L
Up   up down **floor-tap**

Alternate.

Arms shown:
Opposite arm long-lever punching; same arm flexing, elbow kept shoulder high.

Figure 7.68.

Open V-Step

Single lead step, **4 counts.**

R   L   R   L
Up-wide   up-wide   **down-center**   down-center;

This is usually cued: "out", "out", "in", "in".
Arms shown: Same side single bicep curls.

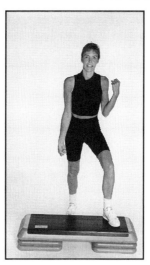

Figure 7.69.

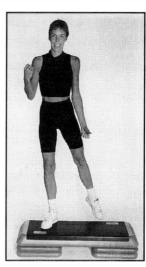

Figure 7.70.

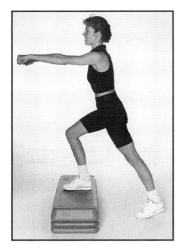

Figure 7.71.

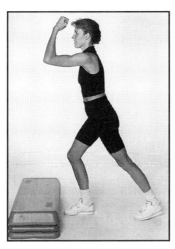

Figure 7.72.

Lunge Backs

Alternating lead step, **8 counts.**

R   L   R   L
Up   up   down   **down and back**

(This is a lunge – no weight bearing.)
Alternate.

Arms shown: Arms punching forward and parallel on up, up; bicep curls keeping elbows still high on the down, down.

▶ STEP-TRAINING BASIC STEP PATTERNS

By-Pass Bench Variations   Figures 7.73–7.76
All are alternating lead steps. 8-count patterns:

Knee-up Bypass

L   R
Up, **knee-lift** (i.e. bypasses the bench and lifts).

     R   L
down (to floor)   down (to floor); Alternate

Arms shown: initiate from arms fully extended out to the sides shoulder high with palms up: Single short-lever curls on the up and knee-lift; return one at a time to the long-lever, shoulder-high initial position on the down, down.

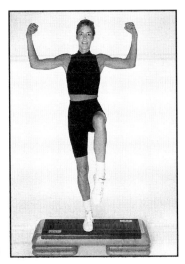

Figure 7.73

Kick Forward By-pass

L   R   R   L
Up **kick forward** down (to floor) down (to floor)

Alternate.

Arms shown: Arms sweep up from sides, together and parallel on up, kick; sweep together and parallel back down to sides on the down, down.

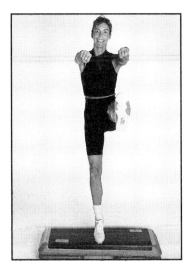

Figure 7.74

Kick-Back By-pass

L   R
Up   **kick back** (a "**long lever** raising" motion)

    R   L
down (to floor)   down (to floor)

Alternate.

Arms shown: initiate from arms fully extended down at sides: Raise same (one) elbow out wide to shoulder high with fist ending at waist, for the up and kick-back; lower to initial position at side with each down, down.

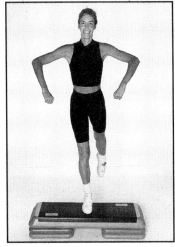

Figure 7.75.

Side Leg-Lift By-pass

L   R
Up **Side leg-lift** (a knee pointing forward position),

    R   L
down (to floor)   down (to floor)

Alternate.

Arms shown: Both arms raised simultaneously to bent-arm lateral raise position for up; same arm (one) extends out to side shoulder high for the side leg-lift; extended arm returns to bent-arm lateral raise on the down; both arms lowered simultaneously on the last down.

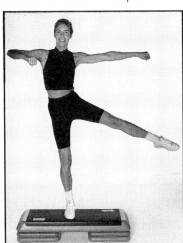

Figure 7.76.

▶ BENCH APPROACH — FROM THE SIDE

Traveling Step — Length of the Bench

Turn Step

A **traveling,** alternating lead step, **8 counts.**

L	R	L	R
Up	**body 1/2 turns left and up**	**down**	**tap-down**

Alternate.

Arms shown: Shoulder-high alternating punch and pull back.

> **Note**
>
> Remember to keep your eyes on the platform. Also, this pattern is shown using natural photography and descriptive words, since it could not be photographed, and therefore described, from a "mirrored" perspective.

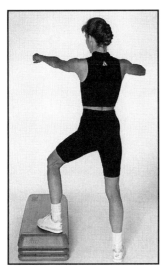 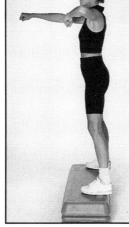 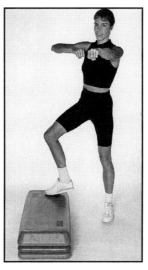 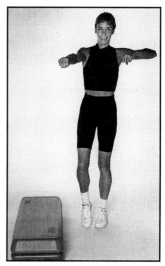

Figure 7.77.	Figure 7.78.	Figure 7.79.	Figure 7.80.

Traveling Step — Width of the Bench

Over The Top

Alternating lead step, **8 counts.**

L	R	L	R
up	**up**	**down on the left side of bench/platform**	**touch-down**

Alternate. Cued: "up", "across","down", "touch-down".

Arms shown: Elbows pointing skyward and shoulder high, with arms wide open on the first, third, fifth and seventh steps; arms low and crossed in front on even-numbered steps.

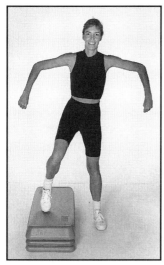 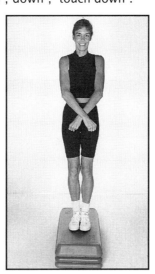 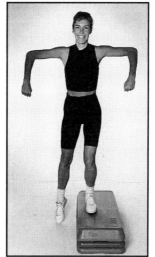 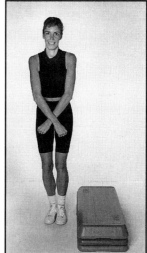

Figure 7.81.	Figure 7.82.	Figure 7.83.	Figure 7.84.

▶ BENCH APPROACH — FROM THE TOP (Facing END of bench)

Straddle Down

Single lead step, **4 counts.**

R
Straddle Down (on R side of bench)

L
Straddle down (on L side of bench)

R   L
Up   Up   **Reverse.**

Arms shown: Shoulder high, short-levers, and fists together at center. Same long-lever arm extends out to side as same leg steps out. One arm at a time returns back in to center on each up, up step.

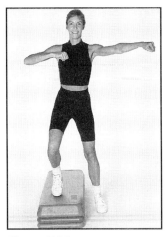

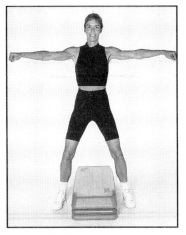

Figure 7.85.   **Figure 7.86.**

▶ BENCH APPROACH — FROM ASTRIDE (straddling bench; see Figure 7.86)

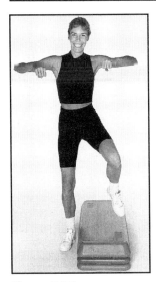
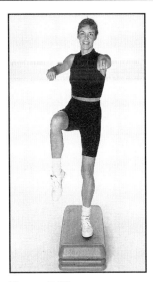

Figure 7.87.   **Figure 7.88.**

Straddle Up By-pass

Alternating lead step, 8 counts.

R   L
Up   **knee-lift** (by-passes bench and lifts waist-high),

L   R
straddle down (to floor)   straddle down (to floor).

Alternate pattern, stepping now up (L) and knee-lifting (R), followed by the straddle down, down.

Arms shown: Same initial position as last pattern, with opposite arm punching forward on lift.

Note:

For variety, try the other by-pass moves shown earlier—kick forward, kick-back, or side leg-lift, incorporating an accompanying arm movement(s) that will keep your balance atop the bench.

▶ STEP PATTERN VARIATIONS[8]   Figures [7.77–7.80]; 7.89–7.96

The following add more variety to the basic step patterns just described and illustrated.

Traveling Steps   (see Figures 7.77–7.80)

An alternating 8 count step pattern, approached diagonally from your front (see Figure 7.52) or your side (see Figure 7.77), using the entire length of the platform, and usually incorporating a partial turning of the body, as you continue to move, either across the bench, or across the floor and bench.

Repeaters

Any alternating 8 count step pattern, in which the **non-weight bearing moves are repeated.**

For example: Using a diagonal front approach, step up, tap up, tap down and back, tap up, tap down and back, tap up, step down (R), step down (L) squarely facing the front of the bench. Alternate stepping up (R) and tapping (L).

For variety, instead of taps use knee-lifts, forward kicks, kick-backs, side leg-lifts, etc.

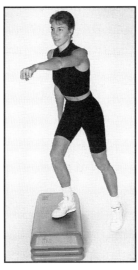 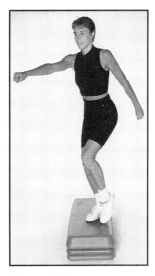 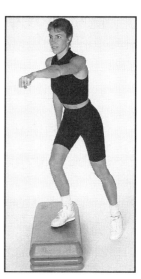

Figure 7.89.   **Figure 7.90.**   **Figure 7.91.**

From the End

You create an 8 or 16 count step pattern that incorporates the use of **all three sides** of the bench, beginning from the end of the bench. Remember, when you get creative, **do not have your back ever facing the bench** while stepping up and down. Therefore, only three sides of the bench are available to you, for any one pattern.

Steps **From The End** use multiple bench-approaches and multiple basic step patterns. Try this sample pattern and then continue on with creating your own patterns, From The End! Chart 15 in the Appendix entitled, "Creating Your Own Step Training Pattern Variations and Aerobic Exercise Routines", is provided for your convenience.

Figure 7.92 illustrates an empty bench with sequential placement location of each foot. Beginning from the bench's end and with your weight on your **right foot** on the floor, step up on bench to the number one #1 location with your **left** foot. Continue on with the pattern, placing your next foot atop/on the side/or at the end - on the floor, wherever the sequential number indicates for foot placement.

Note

When alternating the pattern, final step #16 is a step (taking weight onto L foot). The next move is Up (R).

And, when changing to creating a totally new pattern, final step #16 is a non-weight bearing move (like a "tap"), with the next weight-bearing step on that same ("tap") foot, either in place on the floor, or up, on the bench.

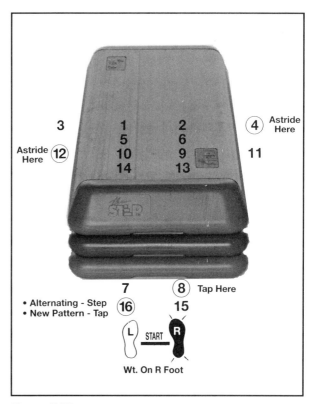

Figure 7.92.

▶ INTERMEDIATE/ADVANCED STEP PATTERNS

Note

During high impact step patterns, (i.e., you are airborne during a portion of the pattern), hand-held weights are not used for safety reasons.

Propulsion Steps

Both feet push off the ground or bench, exchanging positions during the airborne phase of the pattern. Propulsion steps are commonly used with tap and lunge steps.[9] A sample propulsion step pattern is shown in Figures 7.93–7.95. **4 counts.**

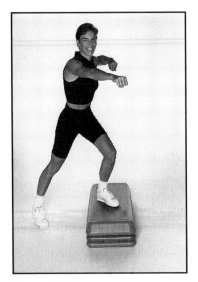

Figure 7.93.
  R   L
Up   **lunge down and back**
2 counts.

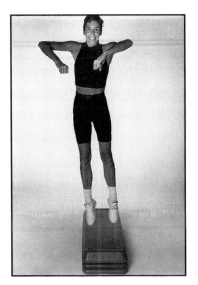

Figure 7.94.
  R
Push off   (with propulsion into this
airborne position).
1 count.

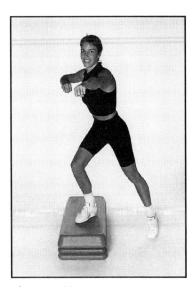

Figure 7.95.   L
Landing on the opposite foot up, then other foot (R) **lunging down and back.   2 counts.**

Step pattern total: **4 counts.**

Adding Hand-Held Weights To Step Training[10]

Extensive criteria for using hand-held weights are given in Chapter 4. **Once you are proficient at stepping**, adding 1-4 lb. hand-held weights can add intensity and variety to your program. The key to adding hand-held weights to step training is maintaining excellent body positioning throughout and being in absolute control of the weights for all upper body movement gestures. Firm "strength/weight training" type arm movements like long-lever raises and/or short-lever curls, symmetrical or in combination as shown in Figure 7.96, are the type of arm movements used for stepping, rather than the more fluid, free-flowing gestures used in aerobics.

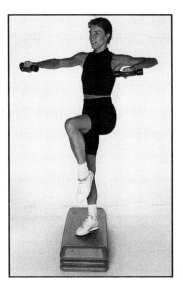

Figure 7.96.

Summary — Step Training Techniques

Techniques illustrating the fundamentals of step training presented here included the following:

▶ Methods to directionally approach the bench.

▶ Understanding correct step training postures, to avoid injuries.

▶ The basic step movements.

▶ The techniques for varying the basic step movements.

As you advance in your fitness and stepping skills, adding variety will become your next challenge, not only by developing more intricate foot patterns, but also by adding many powerful arm movements, taken primarily from strength training principles. And Chapter 8, detailing the principles of choreography, will challenge your creative potential for putting unique possibilities together, after following a few safety guidelines.

Potential and possibilities for using the step-bench do not stop with just aerobic step training, however. It's unique versatility can extend into all of the final or initial segments of your total fitness program hour, as you will soon experience. In order to encourage your exploring the use of this very versatile yet inexpensive piece of equipment in conjunction with the final segments of your aerobics class workout, the exercise techniques presented for the final two program segments will center around using this exciting new equipment phenomenon!

Note

As you will remember, directly preceding the strength training segment and/or stretching and relaxation that is next, will be several minutes of transitional cool-down movement. This primarily serves to slow down the pulse, breathing, and other physiologies which have just been working quite intensely. Be sure that time is taken to make this transition before implementing the strength training and/or stretching segments. You can accomplish this transition with the step-bench by performing a variety of big arm gestures with slow, bench-tapping types of moves.

III. THE STRENGTH TRAINING SEGMENT

Note

The strength training segment is optional in the aerobics class setting, but since it is a vital component of your total physical fitness well-being, most aerobics classes today include from 10–20 minutes of strength-training, in order to provide a well-balanced and complete fitness program. Guidelines from the American College of Sports Medicine state that, "strength training of a moderate intensity, sufficient to develop and maintain fat-free weight, should be an integral part of an adult fitness program. One set of eight to twelve repetitions, of eight to ten exercises that condition the major muscle groups, at least two days per week, is the recommended minimum."[11] Thus, the "prescription" for more fully developing your lean (fat-free) weight is:

Strength Training

Set	Reps	Varieties of Exercises	Minimum Days/Week
1	8–12	8–10 targeting major muscle groups	2 (with max.: 4/week, or every other day)

You can continue to enjoy using the step bench for the strength training segment, focusing on the following isolated muscle groups of the upper, mid, and lower body.

▶ Upper body> chest, upper back, shoulders, and arms.
▶ Mid section> abdominals, lower back.
▶ Lower body> hips and buttocks, thighs, and lower legs.

Techniques presented here use the following types of weight resistance modes:

▶ Commercial rubber resistance bands.
▶ Commercial rubber resistance tubing alone, or with the aid of the bench.
▶ Gravity-assisted techniques, in which the bench is placed in an incline or decline position, with 1–4 pound* hand-held weights, resistance tubing, or using your own body weight as the sole resistance used.

*Note

The bench is not designed for using free-weights that weigh over ten pounds.[12] And, for comfort and safety, place a towel on the bench platform when lying on it.

You'll notice the exercises illustrated and described here have been categorized according to the location of the muscle group(s) benefited (upper body/mid section/lower body) using a variety of equipment means aforementioned. Figure 7.97 illustrates the major muscle groups[13] to be strength trained, and Table 7.1 identifies then, the exercises that will accomplish the training.

Table 7.1. Strength Training Exercises Using Various Forms of Resistance[14,15,16]

UPPER BODY
Chest/Upper Back/Shoulders/Arms

▶ Chest (Pec) Cross-Over
▶ Bent-Arm Chest Cross-Over
▶ Seated Lat Row
▶ Lat Pull Down
▶ Deltoid Lateral Raise
▶ Deltoid Press Away
▶ Deltoid Lateral Raise with Squat
▶ Upright Row
▶ Bicep Curl with Squat
▶ Bicep Curl
▶ Tricep Kick (Press) Back
▶ Overhead Press

MID-SECTION
Abdominals/Low Back

▶ Gravity-Assisted Curl-Up with Weights
▶ Reverse Curl-Up
▶ Back Extension

LOWER BODY
Hips & Buttocks/Thighs/Lower Legs

▶ Buttocks/Heel Lift
▶ Side Leg Raise
▶ Inner Thigh Lift
▶ Leg Curl
▶ Seated Lower Leg Flexor and Extensor
▶ Heel Raise with Squat

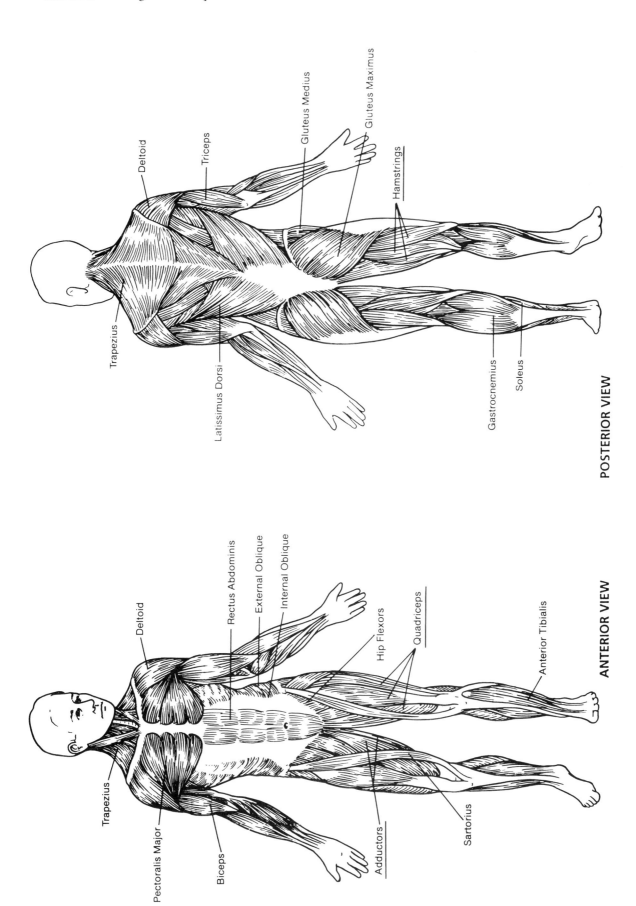

Redrawn from F. D. Giddings, 1980

MUSCLE STRUCTURE[13]

POSTERIOR VIEW

- Deltoid
- Triceps
- Gluteus Medius
- Gluteus Maximus
- Hamstrings
- Trapezius
- Latissimus Dorsi
- Gastrocnemius
- Soleus

ANTERIOR VIEW

- Deltoid
- Rectus Abdominis
- External Oblique
- Internal Oblique
- Hip Flexors
- Quadriceps
- Anterior Tibialis
- Trapezius
- Pectoralis Major
- Biceps
- Adductors
- Sartorius

Figure 7.97. The major muscles to be strength-trained.

▶ UPPER BODY — CHEST ▪ UPPER BACK ▪ SHOULDERS ▪ ARMS

Chest (Pec) Cross-Over

TUBING   (Pectorals)

Position: Step on tubing with one or both feet, with slight bend in knees. Arms are away from body, in front of thighs, no tension.

Action: Cross arms at midline, wrists locked, elbows bent.

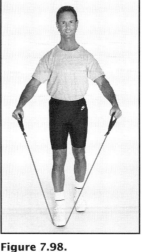
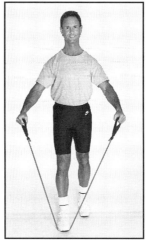

Figure 7.98.   **Figure 7.99.**

Bent-Arm Chest Cross-Over

BENCH AND TUBING   (Pectorals)

Position: Sit center, move buttocks to lower third of bench, lie with head resting at top.

Grab tube under platform at top block where it is grooved. Feet flat on floor, knees in open position.

Action: Cross-punch arm position over chest.

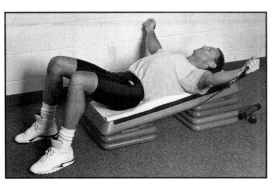

Figure 7.100.

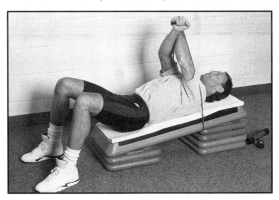

Figure 7.101.

Seated Lat Row   TUBING   (Lats/Trapezius/Rear Deltoid)

Remember, strength training is for women, as well as men, to define and tone lean weight!

Position: Seated, with both knees bent, toes pointed forward, abdominals contracted (to protect lower back). Hands at waist level, fists facing, arms away from body.

Action: Pull elbows behind body, fists facing sides; keep head and spine stationary.

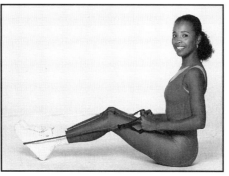

Figure 7.102.

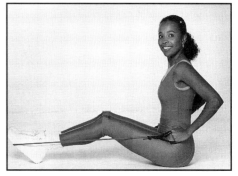

Figure 7.103.

▶ UPPER BODY — CHEST ▪ UPPER BACK ▪ SHOULDERS ▪ ARMS

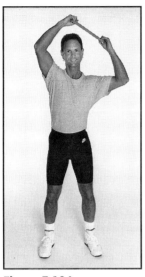 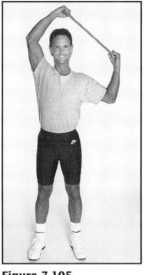

Lat Pull Down

BAND (Latissimus Dorsi)

Position: Grasp band with L hand and place overhead. L elbow is slightly bent, and band is anchored above/behind center of your head.

Action: Grasp band with R hand, keeping hand away from R ear, slowly pull down so R elbow comes into R side of body. Control the return.

Figure 7.104.   **Figure 7.105.**

Deltoid Lateral Raise

BAND (Deltoids/Trapezius)

Position: Grasp band with L hand and anchor it on R hip/side/thigh. Grasp band with R hand, firm fist facing side, elbow bent.

Action: Pull slowly out wide to shoulder height.

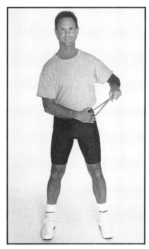 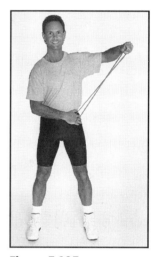

Figure 7.106.   **Figure 7.107.**

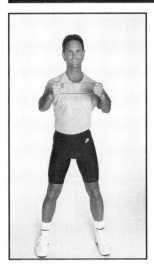 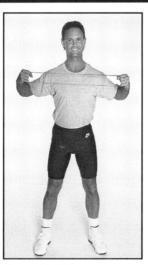

Deltoid Press Away

BAND (Rear Deltoid)

Position: Grab band with both hands, thumbs on top securing band. Arms lower than shoulder height, hands higher than elbows.

Action: Press (pull) hands apart, keeping them directly over elbows. Control return, always keeping it below shoulder height.

Figure 7.108.   **Figure 7.109.**

▶ UPPER BODY — CHEST ▪ UPPER BACK ▪ SHOULDERS ▪ ARMS

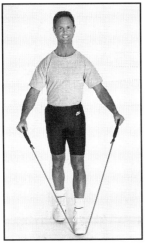
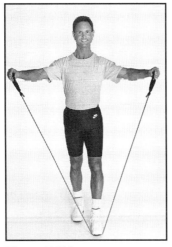

Figure 7.110.   **Figure 7.111.**

Deltoid Lateral Raise

TUBING   (Deltoids/Trapezius)

Position: Step on tubing with R foot, while L foot is behind and L of midline, knees and elbows slightly bent.

Action: Raise elbows away from sides up to shoulder-level while keeping wrists/forearms locked, and hands slightly higher than elbows.

Deltoid Lateral Raise with Squat

BENCH AND TUBING   (Deltoids/Trapezius)

Position: Stand on top of bench with tubing under center, having a fists top/thumbs in and down position.

Action: Press up, bending knees, with hands leading, going only to shoulder level or lower. If fatigued, arms just raise half way.

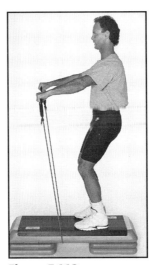
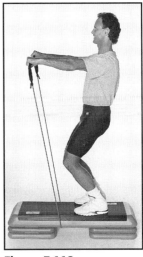

Figure 7.112.   **Figure 7.113.**

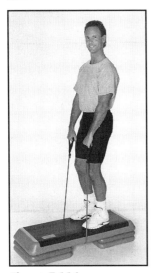
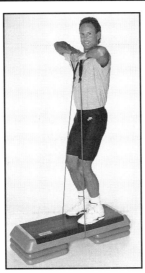

Figure 7.114.   **Figure 7.115.**

Upright Row

BENCH AND TUBING   (Deltoids/Trapezius)

Position: Initial foot and tubing position same, hands/fists now facing and resting on thighs.

Action: Raise handles up to chin, flaring elbows out slightly, keeping spine firmly erect.

Note

Bent knees in all of these illustrations assist in keeping a target heart rate, so that these exercises can also serve as one minute strength training "intervals" in aerobic step training with strength programs.

▶ BICEP CURLS

Bicep Curl with Squat

BENCH AND TUBING   (Bicep/Brachialis)

Position: Same standing, tube location, and hand/fist position facing thighs.

Action: Curl up to sky, rotating palms on the way up so that they face shoulders. Reverse rotation for return. Again, bend knees on the action to increase heart rate.

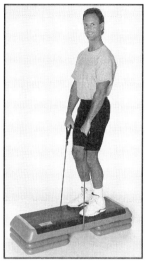 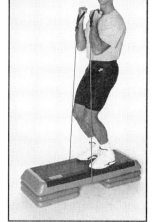

Figure 7.116.   **Figure 7.117.**

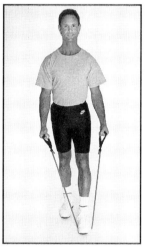 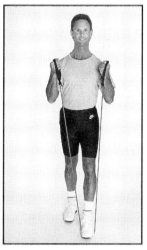

Figure 7.118.   **Figure 7.119.**

Bicep Curl

TUBING   (Biceps/Brachialis)

Position: Step on tubing with one/two feet slight bend in knees, and fists/palms facing body, wrists locked, elbows kept at sides throughout.

Action: Curl both arms toward shoulders.

Bicep Curl

BAND   (Biceps)

Position: L hand anchors band on L thigh. Grasp band with R hand, keeping wrist locked, and R elbow against side.

Action: Curl arm up past chest, wrist ending center and toward R shoulder.

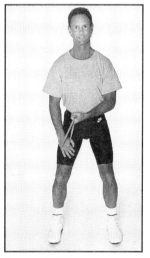 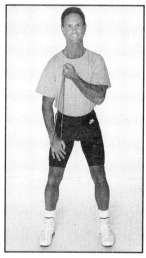

Figure 7.120.   **Figure 7.121.**

▶ TRICEPS

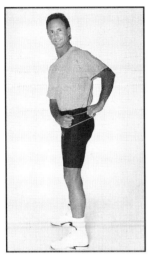 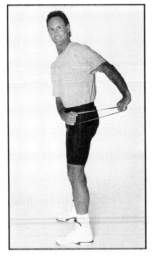

Figure 7.122.   **Figure 7.123.**

Tricep Kick (Press) Back

BAND   (Triceps)

Position: Grasp band with L hand and anchor it on R thigh. Grasp band with R hand, palm/fist facing backward, relaxed position. L arm bent and stabilized against body.

Action: Press arm back to fully extended position. Maintain a good body position.

Tricep Kick (Press) Back

TUBING   (Triceps)

Position: Stand in forward/back stride position, grasp handles with palms facing up/in, elbows "cocked."

Action: Press both arms backward, rotating wrists so palms are facing rear, firm wrists, arms fully extended.

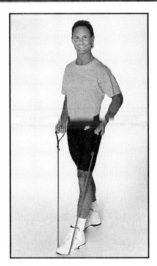 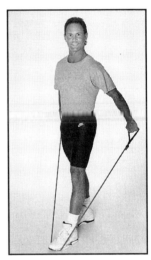

Figure 7.124.   **Figure 7.125.**

Overhead Press

INCLINE BENCH AND TUBING   (Deltoids/Triceps)

Adjust bench so two blocks are at low end and four blocks are at high end.

Position: Prone, with tubing in back of second block's groove, hands starting at sides, wide, and chin resting on incline bench top.

Action: Press up and forward, ending with thumbs in, and facing each other.

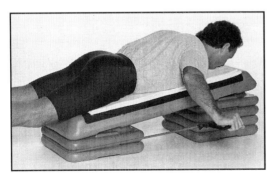 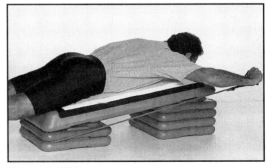

Figure 7.126.   **Figure 7.127.**

▶ MID-SECTION — ABDOMINALS ▪ LOW BACK

Gravity-Assisted Curl-Up

INCLINE BENCH AND 1–4 LB. WEIGHTS   (Abdominals)

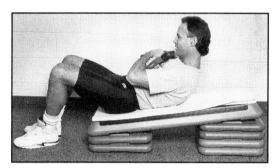

Figure 7.128.

Position: With bench in incline position, straddle and sit on the lower third. Place 1–4 pound free-weights* on sternum (breastbone), with knees flared out wide and heels together, flat on floor. (This leg position works the abdominals.)

Action: Keeping lower back on bench at all times, curl-up, head looking forward. This is all the farther you go; release and curl back down to lying position.

*It is optional to add more weight resistance, but if you do, this is where it should be done.

Reverse Curl-Up

DECLINE BENCH

(Abdominals)

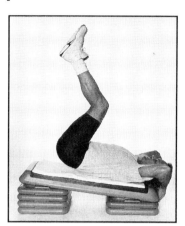

Figure 7.129.

Position: Place bench in a decline position, lie on bench, face up with head at lower end of bench. Grasp lip of platform and top block over your head. Legs are skyward, with hips, knees, and ankles softly bent.

Action: Contract abdominals and raise buttocks up, keeping lower back on the platform. Lower. Remember to evenly breathe on all strength training exercises. It's never acceptable to hold your breath and turn red—your working muscles constantly need oxygen.

Note:

Reps for abdominal work can be 15–30, and 2 sets—one before an aerobics session and one after, because the type of muscle tissue located here responds well to more repetitions for "definition" than other groups of the body. These exercises are to help strengthen "sensitive" lower backs; the low back is completely supported during the abdominal contraction.

Back Extension

INCLINE BENCH   (Erector Spinae)

Position: Lie prone, with hips on lower third, legs extending off bench, supported by toes on floor. With chin on bench, place hands at hips area.

Action: Contract low back and raise upper chest up; hands may move in a sliding motion backward. Lower.

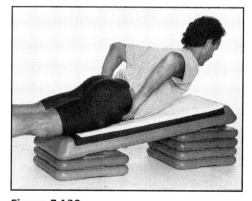

Figure 7.130.

► LOWER BODY — HIPS & BUTTOCKS ▪ THIGHS ▪ LOWER LEGS

Buttocks/Heel Lift

BAND (Gluteals)

Position: Assume an all-fours position, resting on forearms, knees wider than hips, abdominals tight. Place band around L ankle and R instep.

Action: Bend R leg with heel pointing to ceiling, lifting heel without bending knee any further, going as far as band will allow. Lower. Alternate legs, so balance is achieved.

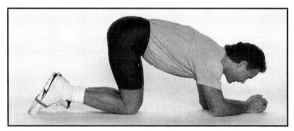

Figure 7.131.

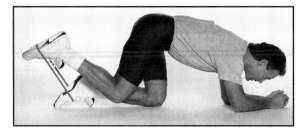

Figure 7.132.

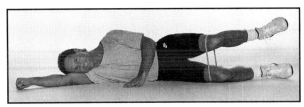

Figure 7.133.

Side Leg Raise

BAND (Thigh Abductors)

Position: Place band just above knees. Lie on side, with head resting on bottom arm which is straight overhead. Top arm is in a bent-arm support in front of chest, with legs either slightly bent or knees bent to 90 degrees.

Action: Raise top leg (bent as shown) 6–12 inches, toward ceiling. Control body position during raising and lowering. After reps, change position and alternate, so both legs are strengthened.

Inner Thigh Lift

BAND (Thigh Adductors)

Position: Lie on side with band placed around instep of both feet. Cross top leg forward, over bottom leg, placing foot flat on floor.

Action: Lift bottom leg up toward ceiling as far as you can, with toes slightly higher than heel. Lower leg slowly, not allowing it to touch floor. Alternate legs after reps completed.

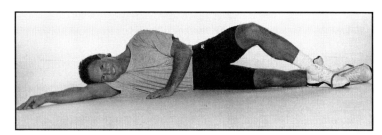

Figure 7.134.

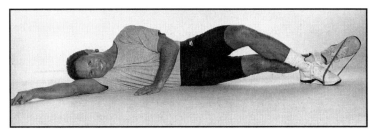

Figure 7.135.

▶ LOWER BODY — HIPS & BUTTOCKS ▪ THIGHS ▪ LOWER LEGS

Leg Curl

BAND
(Hamstrings)

Position: Lie face down, with band around ankles.

Action: Bend R leg, bringing heel toward and within 12–18 inches of buttocks, keeping hips down firmly on the floor. Return. Alternate.

Note: An excellent exercise for the Quadriceps, as a balance to this exercise, is shown in Chapter 4, Figure 4.37. Hips are again held firmly on the floor, and the action alternated after the reps, for balance.

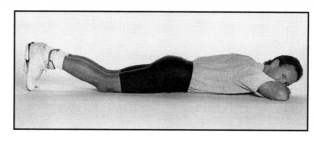

Figure 7.136.

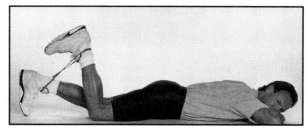

Figure 7.137.

Seated Lower Leg Flexor and Extensor

TUBING   (Tibialis Anterior)

Position: Sit tall, chest raised, shoulders down, holding handles near thighs, palms down, with the tubing around the ball/toe area of both feet held close together.

Action: Without moving body or hands, point toes away from you.

Action: Now, without moving body or hands, point toes toward you, flexing ankles. This is a great exercise for "shin-splints" prevention or relief.

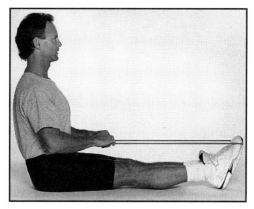

Figure 7.138.

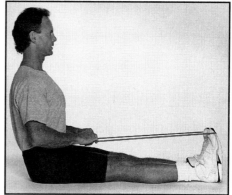

Figure 7.139.

Heel Raise with Squat

BENCH AND TUBING

(Gastrocnemius/Soleus)

Position: Feet center, standing tall. Tubing is placed under center of bench, and held at sides of hips.

Action: Keeping palms stationary (they do not move) at sides, raise heels up, contracting calves ("squeeze"). Lower back down and bend knees. Maintain excellent body alignment.

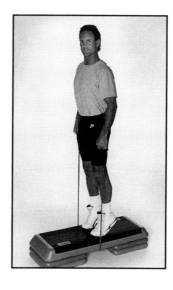

Figure 7.140.

Summary

This concludes an exciting variety of strength training possibilities for you to try. A variety of equipment has been shown training the various muscle groups so that whatever is your preference, or is available to you, you have at least one way to strength train each muscle group. (Even while you are traveling, you can easily pack the light resistance bands or tubing and continue your program uninterrupted.)

Chart 14 in the Appendix entitled, "Strength Training, Using Bands, Tubing, 1–4 lb. Hand-Held Weights, and the Bench" is provided for you to record the following:

▶ The specific exercise techniques you choose for your program.
▶ The number of sets and reps of each exercise you perform.
▶ The types of weight resistance used.
▶ The date of the workout.

Recording your strength training progress, using a variety of equipment choices, will prove to be a very motivational "blueprinting" tool for you to continue on with your program after the formal structure of an aerobics class-setting ends.

IV. COOL-DOWN, FLEXIBILITY TRAINING, AND RELAXATION SEGMENT

▶ COOL-DOWN

Figures [4.41] 7.141

Note

The purpose of a planned cool-down is to give your body time to readjust back to the pre-activity state in which you began. According to whether you have just finished aerobics (exercise or step training), or the optional strength training segment, the time may vary as to how long this transitional cool-down will require. Give yourself time to readjust your pulse, breathing, and other physiologies. Research tells us that the highest incidence of problems occur after an intense workout, so be sure to take this needed time (five minutes minimum) to readjust. Movements are of a step-touch or wide-stride nature, with arms changing from big moves to decreasingly smaller type moves (Figure 7.141).

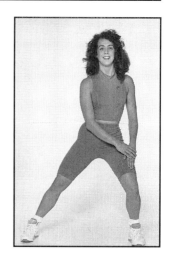

Figure 7.141.

▶ FLEXIBILITY TRAINING

Figures [4.2–4.4; 4.20–4.22; 4.42–4.43; 7.3–7.10] 7.142–7.145

Note

Stretching to increase your flexibility and range of motion is crucial now. It is a time when your muscles are warm (i.e., full of blood, oxygen, and nutrients) and your joints are pliable from vigorous exercise, so take full advantage of the next five to ten minutes to static (or PNF) stretch. Numerous exercise techniques have been presented earlier. Refer to any of these figures to incorporate into your stretching program. Or experiment on the step bench and try the following stretches.

Back Stretch

Sit on the end of the bench with your feet together on the floor. Bend over, resting your chest on thighs. Reach under legs with arms, grasp the opposite elbow and pull both elbows together. Hold.

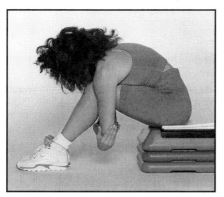

Figure 7.142.

Pectoral Stretch

Lie down on the platform with head and buttocks both comfortably on bench. Press the low back into the bench and place arms out wide to the sides, shoulder level, and palms up. Relax arms as their weight falls toward the floor. Hold.

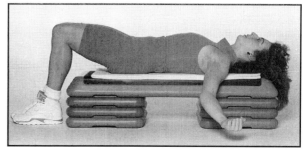

Figure 7.143.

▶ FLEXIBILITY TRAINING

Hamstring Stretch

Still lying on the bench, extend the L leg straight out along the platform, and place foot flat on floor. Grasp behind the R thigh and gently pull the R leg toward the chest. Hold.

Ankle Circling: During the hamstring stretch, slowly circle the foot in all directions. Alternate with L leg and foot.

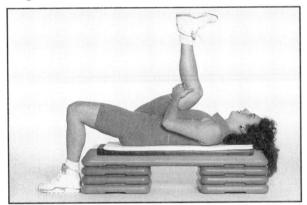

Figure 7.144.

Achilles/Calf Stretch

From the hamstring stretch, pull R knee to chest. Grasp R toes with the hands, and gently pull. Hold. Alternate with L leg and foot.

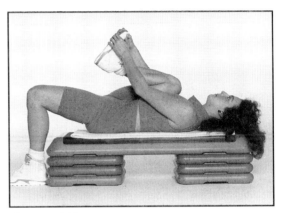

Figure 7.145.

▶ STATIC STRETCHING WITH RELAXATION   Figures [4.44] 7.146

At the conclusion of your workout hour, enjoy the "natural high" your beta endorphins are giving you and begin relaxation techniques in the final stretching segment you perform.

This is the key time to develop rich images and affirmations for yourself, starting with your energized muscles now becoming "wider-and-longer-and-warmer-and heavier". Your breathing is sequential with the pictures and affirmations. Breathe in deeply for 8 counts, hold the breath, and exhale and stretch (Figure 7.146) for 16 counts.

A complete program of relaxation techniques is presented in Chapter 9 to finalize your total physical fitness workout hour.

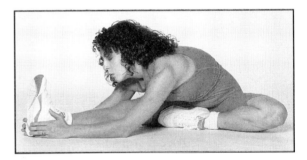

Figure 7.146.

SUMMARY
PROGRAM TECHNIQUES

This chapter, "Start To Finish," has given you a basic blueprint of possible techniques to use for each of the four segments of an aerobics program. You'll next learn how to use these basic moves to create a lifetime of unlimited possibilities, as you try your skills at choreography!

Chapter 8

Choreography: Developing Your Own Program

THE BLUEPRINT FOR UNLIMITED POSSIBILITIES

Choreography is defined as the art of designing or planning movements.[1] Program development principles for choreographing aerobics and step training can be metaphorically compared to the steps used to make a classic, time-honored recipe which is actually just a plan or strategy. A time-honored recipe uses several consistent factors in order to achieve the same excellent results that can be duplicated over and over again by anyone. These consistent factors are: the individual *ingredients* (key components), the *amounts* of each ingredient, and the *order* in which they are best used.

For choreography, you need to understand the key ingredients or the basic components to consider for a balanced program, the amounts that consist of both the variety of movement possibilities available and repetitions of those moves, and the order of their importance (methodology). This constitutes the recipe or blueprint for unlimited movement possibilities! The goal of this chapter is for you to become aware of these three consistent factors (*ingredients/amounts/ order*) so that you can become the creative source of your own personal program or for use when you are placed in the leadership role of directing others.

The Key Ingredients for Balanced Choreography

In both aerobics and step training, exercise movements are pre-planned around these three[2] required key ingredients:

1. to satisfy the need for *biomechanical safety*, so injuries are avoided;

2. with *physiological considerations* in mind, in order to consistently achieve the overall training effect and other individual fitness goals you've set;

3. and *psychologically*, to achieve both short term present-moment enjoyment, and long term enjoyment for program-adherence.

Freestyle choreography or spontaneous improvisation workouts happen when you have advanced to the point where all the principles of biomechanical safety, physiological intensity, and psychological pleasure elements have been permanently set in your mind and are mastered (blueprinted). These principles have become automatically factored into your planning ability, which is then expressed, moment-by-moment, as directed creative movement, coming spontaneously from your internal cueing resources.

Pre-Planning Considerations

The following are some of the main variables considered when pre-planning a well-balanced exercise program which takes into account the key ingredients.

Floor Surface

For aerobics, wood floors are your first choice. Carpeted surfaces will limit your lateral moves and will eliminate all pivoting moves (for knee safety). Avoid concrete surfaces since there is no *give* with impact. If concrete is absolutely the only floor surface available to you, use only low impact and non-locomotor (total body gesturing/no-impact) type of moves. For step training, be sure the floor surface is non-skid or that your bench has provisions for staying in place.

Fitness Level and Motor Skills of the Person(s)

Are the participants:

▶ novices to the activity?

▶ beginners in fitness level or motor skills?

▶ intermediates who are physically fit but have to master some of the basic motor skills involved?

▶ intermediates with excellent motor skills and know a lot of techniques but need to presently become more physically fit?

▶ advanced in both physical fitness and motor skills?

Considerations here are the choice of music tempo (speed) and how you cue and perform the movement — much slower in both regards for the novice and the beginner.

Gender of Participants and Former Movement Experience

Is the group for which this choreography is being planned composed of men, women, or a mixed combination? Do they have athletic/strength training, or performance dance backgrounds? These are especially important to consider when planning the gestures to be used. The small distance between the wrist and the fingertips can be the difference between who participates in your program. Many men overwhelmingly prefer a fist or blade for most hand/palm gestures (Figure 8.1)[3] for both aerobics and step training, and seem to shy away from these activities

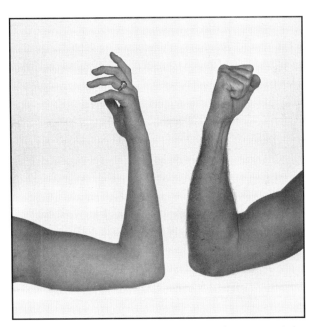

Figure 8.1. The small distance between the wrist and the fingertips can be the difference between who participates in your program and who does not.

if free-flowing performance dance hands are demonstrated or emphasized. Because this is not performance-oriented, but exercise-oriented, you may want to structure all tension-filled hand/palm movements for these activities.

Time-Frame Available

Knowing how much time the participants have, will help to determine how long to make each of the various program segments and whether you can add the fun, extra options, such as relaxation therapy.

Themes

Coordinating special themes and holidays with all phases of your program can be the motivating,[4] psychological boost your participants need every once in a while. It can be carried out in the music you choose, exciting and inviting decorations for the facility, or you can request that participants come dressed uniquely (but safely to perform), or wearing a hat or unique head gear to follow the theme for the day. Or perhaps using a new piece of equipment during the workout (balls, jump ropes, bands, tubing, etc.) will be just the variety needed to keep everyone's spirits uniquely motivated that day.

Intensity of Moves

For aerobics, if you follow the design of the detailed segments given earlier, you'll be able to keep the pulse safely in the training zone during the aerobic segment, and then lower during the warm-up, cool-down, strength training, and stretching segments. The only additional requirement is that the individuals have the skill of pulse-taking (and later recognize their RPE) and what the monitored pulse reading means, so that they (and not you) are held responsible and accountable for their program safety when it comes to heart-rate intensity. Providing the time to take several readings, having a timepiece from which to count, and perhaps providing a visual with the highlights of pulse taking (10 second numbers to achieve or a control dial with numbers and criteria for RPE) are all part of the pre-planning for the program hour.

Additionally, for step training, continually advising the participants how to raise or lower their own intensity (by adding/subtracting hand-held weights, adjusting the bench height up or down, eliminating complex arm movements, or performing only on the floor or bench taps if it becomes necessary), is a skill you'll want to master. This advising is included during the continual cueing of the exercise movements, especially during long repetitions of movements when continual cueing ceases momentarily. This will require that the individuals become responsible for their own intensity levels and ultimately their fitness gains, which is where the burden of risk should lie in all fitness programs.

Impact of Moves

For biomechanical safety, taking into account what stresses are being repeatedly performed is a key to avoiding unnecessary injuries, especially of the hip, knee, and ankle joint areas. Many times simply using a wide variety of impacts (low/power-low/high/and combination high-low), with specific attention to repetitions of same-stress movements, will do much to lessen the negative stress imposed upon the joints and the attending ligaments, tendons, and musculature. Also, the shift from using mostly high-impact (airborne type moves) towards using predominately low-impact and power low-impact moves where the impact has been lessened because one foot is always grounded, has proven to be the necessary key to incorporate into a safe, long-term program.

And, with the aforementioned points in mind, it becomes immediately apparent why the step training phenomenon is sweeping the aerobics industry with unprecedented fervor! Providing a low-impact workout equal in musculoskeletal stress to a 3 MPH pace walk and yet being able to experience the training effect benefits equal to a 7 MPH run[5] is obviously a terrific combination of safety and efficiency.

Kinesthetically Pleasing Moves

Recall from Chapter 1 that kinesthetic means *internal bodily sensations*, which includes three factors: the emotions, muscle movements, and the touch sense.

Motor move combinations need to feel good to perform. Presenting moves which are intellectually challenging yet easy to follow is the goal to keep interest peaked in all levels of skill. Incorporating smooth transitions from one sequence to another by cueing several beats ahead of time, and giving directional hand/head gestures, all help to make the hour psychologically successful for everyone.

There needs to be attention given to the participant's social needs of community building and to the touch-sense. Occasionally planned contact interaction between participants will serve to satisfy both the touch-sense and community building needs we all have. Group movement patterns among participants who don't know each other are more easily integrated during the initial phases of the workout hour, before profuse sweating begins to occur, and serves to set the stage for a highly motivational, emotion-filled hour!

Pre-planning for the three key ingredients for a balanced choreography will do much to enhance your program. Next comes the expanding-the-recipe

or unlimited possibilities concept for successful choreography, by understanding the amount of ingredients with which to pre-plan, and then the method order in which to use the moves.

Amount = Variety and Repetitions

Return to the metaphor of the classic, time-honored recipe. When you decide to add a change in a recipe, you change several possibilities. Either you increase the same ingredients , such as the repetitions in choreography, or you carefully add favorite new ingredients (variety of moves in choreography) that will work into the basic recipe. Repetitions of moves have been adequately discussed thus far. The remainder of this section will list the basics and then present a variety of possibilities to add to those basics.

Movement Possibilities: The Foundation From Which To Build

Aerobics Impact Moves

The force exerted when the foot contacts the floor)

1 **Low-Impact Movement** (one foot always remains in contact with the floor):

▶ Bouncing Two-Feet

▶ Bounce 'n Hitch-Kick

▶ Bounce 'n Tap Series

▶ Half-Time Galloping

▶ Hoedown

▶ Heel-Toe Bounce Series

▶ Kicking (from ankle/knee/hip)

▶ Knee-Lift Varieties (forward/sideways/across)

▶ Lunging Varieties

▶ Marching

▶ Pace-Walking

▶ Side Step-Out

▶ Step-Touch

2 **Power Low-Impact Movement** (forceful lifting and lowering):

▶ Heel Jacks

▶ Jogs

▶ Two-Foot Jumps

▶ Kicks

▶ Knee-Lifts

▶ Lunging

- ▶ Ponies
- ▶ Step-Touches
- ▶ Twist

3 High-Impact Movement (great force exerted when the foot contacts the floor; controlled landing is important):

- ▶ Galloping
- ▶ Hitch-Kick
- ▶ Hopping Varieties (single, double, with kicks and knee-lifts)
- ▶ Jogging
- ▶ Jumping Varieties (single, stride, widestride or closed, hopscotch)
- ▶ Leaping
- ▶ Polka
- ▶ Prancing
- ▶ Rocking
- ▶ Running
- ▶ Skipping
- ▶ Sliding

Step Training Impact Patterns

Includes all patterns where one foot is always in contact with the bench or floor, or you are momentarily airborne.

1 Low-Impact Basic Step Patterns (one foot should always be in contact with the bench or floor):

- ▶ Basic Bench Step
- ▶ By-Pass Bench Variations (knee-up, kick forward, kick backward, side leg-lift)
- ▶ From the End
- ▶ Lunge Backs
- ▶ Open V-Step
- ▶ Over the Top
- ▶ Repeaters
- ▶ Single Cycle Bench Tap
- ▶ Single Cycle Floor Tap
- ▶ Step Tap
- ▶ Straddle Down
- ▶ Straddle-Up Bypass
- ▶ Turn Step
- ▶ Traveling Steps

2 High-Impact Variation Step Pattern (momentarily airborne):

- ▶ Propulsion Steps

Gesturing

Movement of any non-weight bearing body part (head, shoulders, fingers, hands, arms, torso, one leg, or foot)

1 Basics:

- ▶ Bending
- ▶ Circling
- ▶ Closing
- ▶ Curling
- ▶ Opening
- ▶ Pulling
- ▶ Pushing
- ▶ Shaking
- ▶ Stretching
- ▶ Swaying
- ▶ Swinging Arms/Legs/Torso
- ▶ Tapping
- ▶ Turning
- ▶ Twisting

2 Variations:

- ▶ Different Styles
  - ▶ Athletic-Sports Moves
  - ▶ Classic
  - ▶ Funk
  - ▶ Jazz
  - ▶ Martial Arts
  - ▶ Military
  - ▶ Western
  - ▶ Create your own!
- ▶ Adding Sounds
  - ▶ Claps
  - ▶ Finger Snaps
  - ▶ Slaps (Thigh/Ankles)
  - ▶ Specific Gestures With Audibles (military chants, shooting pistols, contact sounds, popular words and phrases — "Uh-huh")

Adding More Variety to the Basic Steps and Gestures

For both aerobics and step training, the following guidelines apply for adding more variety to your basic foot patterns and gestures.

1 **Vary the Levers:** (Movement initiated from this joint)

▶ Arms
   ▶ From elbows — short lever moves
   ▶ From shoulders — long lever moves

▶ Legs
   ▶ From knees — short lever moves
   ▶ From hips — long lever moves

2 **Vary The Planes and Levels:** Limbs move over and around the body

▶ Planes
   ▶ Horizontal/Vertical/Diagonal

▶ Levels
   ▶ Low (knees), Medium (chest), High (overhead)

3 **Vary the Directionality and Pathways:** Movement that is toward/away from/or turning to face/an external directional point

▶ Directionality
   ▶ Up/Down
   ▶ Right/Left
   ▶ Forward/Backward
   ▶ Diagonal

▶ Pathways
   ▶ Straight (lines/square/dueling sides)
   ▶ Curved (spiral/double circle — same and opposite/two parallel ovals — partners meet and join)
   ▶ Zig-Zag (V path/Z path)

4 **Vary The Rhythm:**

▶ How much movement or how many steps/gestures are performed in a unit of time (movement every beat; movement every other beat; movement at twice the tempo-speed-of the beat).

▶ Which beats are accented in a unit of time (*one*–2–3–4; 1–*two*–3–4; 1–2–*three*–4; 1–2–3–*four*; *one*–*two*–3–4; 1–2–*three*–*four*; *one and two*–3–4; 1–2–*three and four*; *one*–2–*three*–4; 1–*two*–3–*four*; *one*–*two*–*three*–*four*!)

5 **Vary The Symmetry:**

▶ Perform symmetrical movement (arms/legs/arms and legs/performing the same movement, at the same time).

▶ Perform asymmetrical movement (arms/legs/arms and legs/performing in opposition to one another).

6 **Vary the Force (of Impacts and Gestures):**

▶ According to:
   ▶ The phase of the program
   ▶ Current fitness levels present
   ▶ Motor skills present

▶ Range of possibilities:
   ▶ No impact with low intensity gestures
   ▶ High impact with high intensity gestures

▶ Under this category, consideration is given to the question, "Should one use hand-held weights for aerobics programs?" Criteria for safely using hand-held weights for aerobics are the following:
   1. *Only* if you are at the *intermediate or advanced physical fitness* and motor skill level.
   2. *Only* if you can maintain *a good body position* (posture) throughout the hour.
   3. **This guideline is of key importance:** Only arm movements and gestures similar to those used for weight training (Figure 8.2) should be performed in aerobics when hand-held weights are

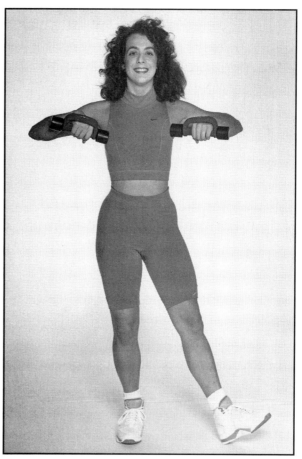

Figure 8.2. Only arm movements and gestures similar to those used for weight training should be performed in aerobics.

added. This means you must maintain absolute control of the range of motion and velocity you use. Hand-held weights cannot safely be used for the fast, flailing movements characteristic in many aerobics programs. Therefore, considerable adaptation on your part must take place in order to safely add hand held weights to the aerobic segment of your aerobics program. The same three guidelines are appropriate for adding hand-held weights when step training. More detailed guidelines are given in Chapter 4 for the use of hand-held weights during step training.

7 Use a Variety of Established Dance Steps and Dances

Note: These are all used very successfully in the aerobics dance-exercise setting. With a little alteration, many of these can also creatively be adapted into the Step Training program. Remember, creativity is unlimited; the only boundaries are safety, suitability, and those you personally impose.

- ▶ Bunny Hop
- ▶ Cha Cha
- ▶ Charleston
- ▶ Grapevine/Stroll
- ▶ Hustle
- ▶ Jitterbug
- ▶ Funk
- ▶ Fox Trot
- ▶ Mexican Hat Dance
- ▶ Polka

Order = Methodology: How and When the Movements Are Put Together in Combinations

The order, or method, of how and when all of the movement possibilities presented in this chapter are put together in combinations is called sequencing. The three variables around which the order of movement is sequenced are the three main ingredients mentioned earlier: biomechanical safety needs, physiological intensity needs, and the psychological needs attendant to a positive, pleasant workout (i.e., intellectually challenging but easy to follow, etc.). Sequencing possibilities are:

1 Continual Progression of Moves: Performing isolated step/gesture movements. For example,

using an alphabet of moves, like (A) arm circles, (B) bouncing and tapping, (C) cross-step and hop, etc.

2 Add On: Linking two moves together, before another is added. You can then continually link, repeating all movement and adding on for a specific time frame. For example, sequence 1; sequence 1, add on 2; sequence 1, 2, add on 3.

3 Pyramid: Progressively more or fewer repetitions of moves or counts of music. For example, moves performed for 4–3–2–1 repetitions; or 1–2–3–4 repetitions. Many times movement transitions execute well if a "hold" move or count is added to the uneven numbered repetitions, so the sequence fits smoothly into four or eight counts of music. The aerobics Bounce 'n Tap Series can be an excellent use of Pyramid sequencing, and can be performed for an entire song, using either low-impact bouncing and directionally tapping, or high-impact hopping and tapping.

4 Patterns: Any two or more combinations of moves repeated in a certain repetitive cycle.

- ▶ This is why the basics for step training are usually described as patterns. Isolated steps can be part of the variety offered, but most of the movement is performed as two or more combinations of moves. Samples: Up, up, down, down; or up, kick, down, tap.

- ▶ Many patterns together would then be present in a routine. Routines are start-to-finish choreographed movement.

SUMMARY

This chapter detailing choreography represents independence to you. It systematically takes apart how movement is safely and efficiently planned, to meet your needs. Chart 15 in the Appendix entitled, "Creating Your Own Step Training Pattern Variations and Aerobics Exercise Routines" has been devised for you to practice choreographing movement for an exercise session. Enjoy the unlimited aerobic movement possibilities that can be performed when mixing and combining the variety of options offered here. There are absolutely no boundaries to creativity!

Chapter 9

Stress Management Principles and Relaxation Techniques

◆ ◆ ◆

UNDERSTANDING "BALANCE" FIRST

Committing yourself to developing the mindset for fitness, or living a total wellness lifestyle in which your stress is managed, or being able to tap into your full, unlimited potential all sound very exciting to achieve. Experiencing personal excellence in any or all of the dimensions of your life requires, at some point, becoming more aware of your potential and unlimited possibilities. To understand potential and possibilities, we must each begin by setting a *standard* (establishing a starting point or basis) from which to grow.

Total wellness, your stress in balance, a balanced state of well-being, or an integrity or wholeness of the mind/body/spirit are ways of expressing this ideal condition we strive to achieve daily. Once we take apart this abstract concept and label its parts, it will become more clear just how to initiate the process. This will then lead to your managing or achieving the most productive and rewarding results imaginable in any and all of the dimensions of your life.

ESTABLISHING THE FOUNDATION

All of our world and universe is based on balance. Personal wellness is your life in balance. It requires actions, emotions, attitudes, beliefs, your will, and your power-source all kept in mind and utilized, when problem-solving.

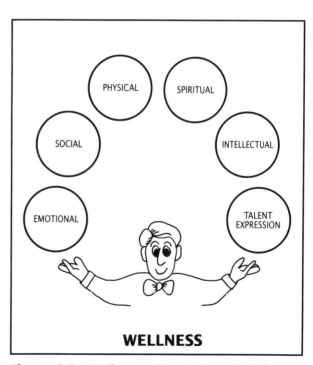

WELLNESS

Figure 9.1. Wellness achieved through balancing six key dimensions of your life.

Life balance or *wellness* is easily understood when pictured as six components or *balls* that we need to keep juggling in the air, all at once. These six components include our physical, emotional, social, spiritual, intellectual, and talent expression well-being. Figure 9.1 depicts a visual model of wellness. It reflects that each of these six components is an equally important contributor, to the total balancing act we must engage in every day.

When any wellness component or ball being juggled and kept in balance gets temporarily overlooked, or forgotten totally, it falls out of this balanced alignment and drops out of sight. We report being *out of sync* with life, or we get the feeling of *not being whole*. This is understandable, because we aren't! We've allowed one or even several of the six components of our lives to take over and receive all of our attention.

For example, if the expression of our talent (our job, or career pursuit, or volunteering) takes an enormous amount of our mental and physical energy every day little time is left to participate in a physical fitness program, to develop a social network of friends, or to intellectually pursue other interests that can provide positive release of our stress. Our physical, social, or intellectual ball drops and is forgotten. We soon experience the results of this choice — a decline in our physical fitness, loss of a well-rounded social network of friends, or a boring one dimensional focus in all of our daily conversations.

SUCCESS

How do we know if and when we have done an excellent job of balancing all of these six areas of our lives? Developing a working definition for *success* — knowing when you've achieved this balance — is one good way. Take some quiet time to develop your own definition for success. A definition for success that works for many people is the following. Try this out to see if it gives you answers to "what is balance in my life?"

You can then unconditionally believe that you have been *successful* in anything you attempt in life if

♦   ♦   ♦

*Success is the ongoing process of
striving and growing to become more,
in each of the dimensions of wellness,
while positively contributing to others' needs.*

♦   ♦   ♦

you have 1) attempted and grown from it; 2) made more distinctions about what you're doing, and 3) accomplished it for the purpose of positively contributing what you've learned to others. Can you see by adopting this definition for success, that it is very difficult to feel like a loser or failure?

Everything described thus far can be accomplished if you think of each as steps in a journey, rather than a destination. Life is an ongoing process, and wellness and success are both landmarks in the journey. Realize early in life that there is no one port or station in life — no one place to arrive at — once and for all. The true joy of life is the trip! A final port or permanent station is a mental image, and is always to be held in expectation, so that our unlimited potential can constantly be tapped to creatively problem-solve. Life must be lived and enjoyed in the present moment as accomplished steps, as we go along. For the final port will come along soon enough.

BALANCING THE SIX WELLNESS DIMENSIONS

Each component or dimension of wellness — each ball we juggle — has specific themes that are explored in this text, either lightly or in-depth. Since the design of *Aerobics ♦ The Way To Fitness* is primarily mastery of physical fitness, more emphasis has, of course, been placed on the details of this wellness component. The other components are addressed in detail throughout the text, where the points are appropriate.

The *Physical Wellness* component reflects having a regular program of the physical expenditure of energy for increasing one's flexibility, heart and lung capacity, and muscular strength and endurance; maintaining a good body position (good posture) while exerting this physical effort; selecting a proper intake, both variety and amount, of food and liquid; and maintaining a proper body weight (lean-to-fat ratio).

Although wellness and fitness are sometimes synonymous terms in various media, the term *fitness* within this text carries a more specific meaning and refers to a measured and quantified degree of a particular wellness component. For example, you exhibit physical fitness if you are a twenty-year-old male and can run/walk 1.5 miles in twelve minutes.[1] The term will reflect a specific result you've achieved by directly measuring it against accepted norms established by the health professional community. Fitness, like wellness and success, is not an end. It must constantly be worked on to keep the standard you've achieved and to realize your full, unlimited possibilities.

The *Emotional Wellness* component reflects obtaining balance in how we deal with pleasure and pain (see Figure 9.2). It takes a look at the distinctions or labels for pleasure (joy) and pain (sadness, anger, fear) and the mixed neuro-associations we feel when these two big emotions are blended (confusion first, then a various assortment and labeling of distinctive others).

Becoming aware of the precise emotions we feel and also being aware of what we link to pleasure and pain, will assist us in being rational and able to choose productive behavioral responses to life situations, when we encounter them.

The *Social Wellness* component involves creating balance in your alone time and need for others time. We can, of course, choose to be independent persons and achieve every goal we ever set alone. But you will soon find out, within the later sections on using the various resources you have, that the most successful and mature persons, who regularly tap into their full, unlimited potential are those persons who are *inter*-dependent people. They choose to use other people on a regular basis, even when they could fully accomplish their goals alone. They are able to stretch themselves to unbelievable heights, because others are constantly used as key resources.

Another important theme in the Social Wellness component is becoming aware of your communication skills. Sharpening both your assertiveness and confrontational skills with others will assist you in becoming a victor, instead of a victim in life.

The *Intellectual Wellness* component challenges you to become a life-long learner, and to never become complacent and satisfied with past learning and accomplishments. Keeping an open mindset to growth and change in the world at large, will help us to realize there are no boundaries to our potential, individually or collectively. The only boundaries, or limits to our potential, are the ones that we self-impose inside our heads. Every chapter of this text holds intellectual wellness ideas to consider — new points to ponder.

The *Spiritual Wellness* component challenges you to investigate the balance that must exist between relying on your own self-energy source (will power), and that which ultimately "fuels" you. Finding purpose or the meaning of your existence is assisted by developing a belief system, expressed as philosophies by which you consistently live your life daily.

The *Talent Expression* component is the sixth dimension of wellness to keep in balance. Your talents are your natural and trained abilities and interests

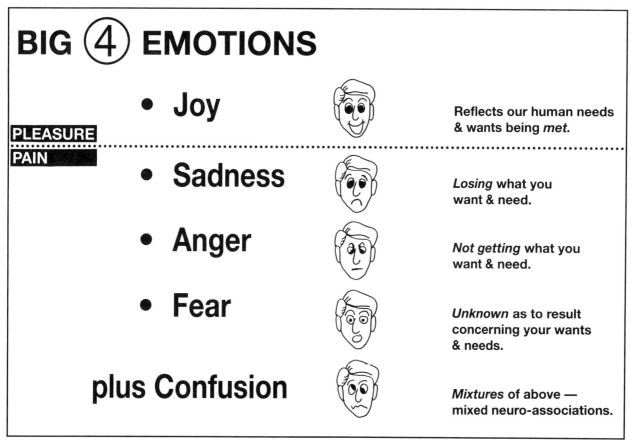

Figure 9.2. The Four Big Emotions.

that become your career path or jobs, the volunteer giving of your time to others, and many times the activities that you engage in to relieve your stress (stress outlets). Because it usually has a significant impact on self-worth and prestige, this is an area that is probably one of the most difficult for us to keep in perspective, and balanced with the other five dimensions of wellness.

OUR FOUR BASIC NEEDS

Why do we want to keep our wellness in balance — for what reasons, purposes, or intentions? There are four clearly defined categories of survival needs that we all must have met, that are supported by the wellness components of our lives:

1. I need to live and be healthy.
2. I need to be loved.
3. I need prestige (self-worth) and power (the ability to take action).
4. I need variety and change in my life.

These needs can be compared to *birthrights* that we all require for survival and should never be taken away or used as avenues by which to manipulate another.

In addition to our four basic needs are our wide variety of wants. Our *wants* are the privileges or extra comforts we attempt to have by being responsible and accountable for the actions we take in life. It is important to not only label what we require for survival (our *needs*, which we also call our ends or ultimate goals), but also what would give us additional pleasure and joy in the process (our *wants*, also called the means to our ends, or our time priorities). Only when we have a clear understanding of both our basic needs and our desires or wants will we have labeled the purposes and intentions for our various wellness decisions.

BALANCE IN BRIEF

The foundation of life is based upon balance or a *wellness state*. This wellness state is comprised of six dimensions — our physical, emotional, social, spiritual, intellectual, and talents expression well-being. Developing an all-encompassing definition for success in life provides us with the opportunity to measure and know if and when we achieve individual life balance, and have kept the six wellness balls juggled. The various themes addressed within each component of wellness covered throughout this text gives a sampling of program ideas on how to develop

exceptionally well in each area. Developing this balance will satisfy both our survival needs and our additional pleasure-filled wants.

It is time to place all of these definitions and concepts into real life problem-solving, and consider: what happens when an imbalancing occurs and stress enters our life? We must be realistic and aware that all of life will not be a continual, perfect balance for us, for life is not static and unchanging. Change is a constant, and the only way for growth to occur is for change to happen. Thus we must consider when this imbalancing enters our life, how do we deal with growth and change?

FROM IMBALANCE TO STRESS/TIME/LIFE MANAGEMENT

Take a long moment to ponder the following. Envision a beautiful, sunny, mid-western late-fall day, and you are standing next to a huge fifty-year-old maple tree, which is completing the process of changing its colors from summer-green to the majestic yellows, oranges, and reds of fall. Having this picture firmly set in your mind, can you now clearly understand the following quote?

It is only through change that we grow.

STRESS: DEFINED AND MANAGED

Demands. Problems. Challenges. Change. Whatever you choose to call it, within the journey of life, *imbalance happens*. We cannot control the changes, demands, problems, or even the dirty deals we experience. We can learn how to manage certain situations so that they are less offensive to us (i.e., use preventive measures), but we cannot control our world and all it presents to us. Drunk drivers permanently injure us. Fire or floods destroy our homes and belongings. Death takes our loved ones. A close friend permanently moves far away. We win the lottery! Imbalance will happen daily and throughout our life, and we are left to react. *Stress* is our response.

Probably the most noted scientific researcher in modern times on the topic of stress and its effect on the human body is the late Viennese-born endocrinologist, Hans Selye. In his words:

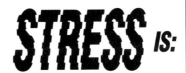

STRESS IS: *The non-specific response of the body to any kind of demand that is made upon it.*

PHYSIOLOGICAL RESPONSES TO STRESS

The physiological response your body exhibits to the positive or negative stressful demands that are made upon it from life situations includes the following:

▶ There is an increase of sugar in the blood.

▶ Your rate of breathing increases.

▶ Your heart rate increases.

▶ Your blood pressure increases.

▶ There is an activation of the blood clotting mechanism to protect you from injury.

▶ There is increased muscle tension.

▶ There is a cessation of digestion, and the blood is diverted to the brain and muscles.

▶ There is increased perspiration output.

▶ There is decreased salivation.

▶ There is a loosening of bladder and bowel muscles.

▶ There is an outpouring of various hormones, like adrenalin.

▶ Your pupils dilate.

▶ And there is a heightening of all of your senses.

In effect, then, your body goes into a "Red Alert" and you are ready to fight or take off (flight). This has thus been named the *fight or flight* response to stress.

Many times you can't do either — fight or flight — and you must stay in the situation and "stew." If this response, as characterized by the above list, is long enough or severe enough, you then experience wear and tear on your bodily systems. This leaves you open to the invasion of some sort of illness.

Once a person becomes ill, the illness also becomes a stressor. This will increase your stress response (again, as described in the list of bodily changes) and you may feel as if you are caught in a double-bind.[3]

So, good or bad, with any kind of imbalancing — demands, problems, challenges, or changes — stress is our response. Therefore, scientifically and physiologically speaking, stress is viewed as a *neutral* term. There is positive stress (called *eustress*) like running a marathon or seeing our loved one after seven months at war, and there is negative stress (called *distress*) like experiencing a car accident or our home being vandalized. The goal with managing either kind of stress is the same as with all of life — to achieve a balanced state. This can be more easily understood using several analogies.

Stress management in our life can be compared to playing a guitar. To play the guitar, we must use strings which come in a package, all limp and with no tension on them (no demands or challenges). We can make no sounds if there is no tension or stress on the strings. The same comparison goes for our lives — if we have no stress, we have no challenges, no risks, no growth. Life is boring and so are we because there is just not enough going on in our life. But stretch those strings to their potential by placing them on the instrument and placing just the right amount of tension on them, add the human touch, and we will experience beautiful sounds — harmony — new possibilities. Place too much tension on the strings (add too many commitments for our time) and even the slightest pressure will cause the strings to pop and so will we.

This same analogy can be used visualizing air within a balloon. If there is no air there is no tension — only a limp existence. The right amount of air and tension in the balloon gives you beauty in all the richest colors life can offer. But too much air — too much tension — too many time commitments in any and all of your wellness areas, and you break! Your life becomes fragmented, disjoined, non-whole.

So in order to experience life with continual growth, imbalance must occur to create room for new unlimited possibilities. Change is one of the certainties of life. It is a given. If we approach change with a positive perspective, it can open the doors to unlimited growth and possibilities. If we take the negative view, and see it as a threat to our comfortable stability, change can imprison us in the depths of despair and result in our stagnation. The choice of perspective, and the subsequent reactions we have, is ours to make.

STRESS/TIME/LIFE MANAGEMENT

Earlier in this chapter, establishing an ideal foundation for our life had us look at balance. Now, with real life situations constantly impacting upon us, we add a dimension to this and consider the role of imbalance in our lives.

The key in understanding both of these concepts is that there is an appropriate time-frame of "how much" and "when" that we must develop the ability to manage for both balance and imbalance. The time-frames we arrive at as we problem solve our life and stress will be unique and different for each one of us.

Have you begun to realize that stress management — managing your response to change — is really life management? And that time management—managing the individual moments of your life — is also life management?

Managing the moments of your life, whatever these moments consist of, is managing your life and therefore managing your self. Holding onto this key thought, you will now commence taking the exciting trip inward, to become consciously aware of what unique resources lie inside of you, just waiting to be tapped and put into action, to achieve personal excellence in your life, every single day!

"To reveal myself openly and honestly takes the rawest kind of courage."[2]

IDENTIFYING YOUR INTERNAL RESOURCES

This is an autobiographical inventory of your wants, needs, and key life experiences. Tapping into your unlimited potential in order to experience balance, the management of your stress, or daily excellence, requires you to take a long moment and look at your six wellness dimensions in terms of the multitude of resources you have experienced or developed in your past and present, and any you've designed for your future. Chart 16 in the Appendix entitled, "Identifying and Fully Using Your Top 20 Resources" is provided for this very unique assessment.

This *resource awareness* exercise will assist you in understanding not only the physical, emotional, physical, spiritual, intellectual, and talent expression wellness points at which you are beginning this personal journey inward, but also will give you the keys to accessing and enhancing your future. It will help you to become aware of your:

▶ hereditary and environmental influences to date;

▶ positive and negative life experiences;

▶ wants, needs, priorities, and goals;

▶ strength, talents, and interests;

▶ weaknesses, risk factors, and poor choices;

▶ thoughts and programming — what is on your mental tapes;

▶ beliefs, truths, and parameters of acceptance:

▶ attitudes, your explanatory life-style;

▶ feelings or emotions; and

▶ behaviors expressed, which result from all of the above.

Whether they are currently interpreted as positive or negative by you, by identifying each of these resources that you have, you'll gain an initial awareness now, and later on insight, into how to use them

effectively to obtain balance, the management of your stress, and daily excellence in many areas of your life. However, it does take risk-taking and vulnerability on your part — a willingness to be open and honest and:

1. A trust that these questions will enable you to view and begin to give meaning to some of your innermost thoughts; and

2. A trust in yourself that you *can* greatly change, improve, stretch yourself, and tap into your full, unlimited potential to manage your stress and problem-solve life's daily challenges.

ASSESSMENT OF YOUR COPING SKILLS

After having taken the resources inventory, you have undoubtedly discovered that you are a person with many resources that are unique to you. Now consider this: How have you chosen to use these resources in the past to cope(regain balance) when life has given you an imbalancing experience?

You're beginning to realize that in order to stay mentally balanced, we all do *something* to cope with the stress in our lives. Some of these coping mechanisms are positive and some of them are detrimental to our total well-being. Located on Chart 17 in the Appendix entitled, "Reflecting Upon Your Stress Outlets" is a list of common coping mechanisms called *stress releases*. Take note as to how you habitually cope with stress, i.e., what your positive means are and what your negative and detrimental means are, and then establish a goal to work on improving the one key response to stress that is most disabling to you.

You will probably come away from this reflection and self-assessment being a lot less judgmental of other people and their abilities to cope with stress. Just knowing that we all do something to relieve and cope with the stress in our lives can help you to tolerate another person's choices that sometimes directly affect you. You come away realizing that some people are not *bad* people, because, say, they smoke cigarettes, but are simply making a *bad choice* in their means of reducing the stress in their lives.

When you are successful in adjusting to and managing your response to stress, it can provide you with growth and an increased confidence for meeting the next challenge (life situation) that comes to you. We each learn how to adjust to the everyday big and small problems and life situations that are presented to us simply by using the vast internal resources we have stored within. We are not born adjusted; we systematically learn our adjustments.

USING YOUR RESOURCES TO MANAGE STRESS

There are many effective strategies that can be learned to manage stress. Developing your ability to relax is among the most important. Here are several guided imagery techniques to use following the positive stress of your workout hour, or to relieve the negative stresses you encounter every day. Each technique takes only a few minutes to visualize. If more than one technique is used at a time, you'll find that they have a *cumulative effect*, and a deeper relaxation will be experienced, perhaps even culminating in sleep.

So choose what result you desire. You may wish to simply enhance a workout with one brief relaxation technique lasting three minutes in order to successfully lower your heart rate and breathing, cease sweating profusely, and curb other physiologies. Or you may want to simply rejuvenate yourself for ten minutes during a busy day by refocusing your attention before a big event such as an exam, speech, athletic contest, or interview, by using two techniques. At bedtime you may choose to totally relax to the point that you go directly to sleep, which may take using just one or all of the techniques.

Two successful methods for using these techniques are:

1. having someone cue you by reading them slowly;

2. recording them slowly onto a cassette tape, and then playing them to relax.

Enjoy these classic guided-imagery techniques and then develop more imagery of your own by using your identified internal resources. Take a trip to your favorite vacation spot or re-experience talking to the heroes and role models in your life.

♦ ♦ ♦

Ease the pounding of your heart by the quieting of your mind.

♦ ♦ ♦

GUIDED IMAGERY

 Total Body Scanning

This technique differs greatly from many other equally effective methods. It utilizes your powers of control through your imagination. Your mind seeks out and recognizes tension. It then eliminates it through your ability to imagine the relaxation. No physical exertion or planned tensing of muscle groups is performed. There are four steps to total

body scanning: establishing the position; establishing the breathing pattern; tuning in to various parts of the body; and a heart rate monitoring followed by simple static stretching to make you alert again, unless the technique is used prior to going to sleep.

Step I: Relaxation Position

▶ Lie on your back (Figure 9.3). If you feel uncomfortable because your entire back is not in contact with the floor raise one knee up with your foot flat on the floor approximately one foot from your buttocks (Figure 9.4). Persons with either substantial buttocks or shoulder mass will find that this "knee up" position will relieve the arched lower back feeling.

▶ Turn your head slightly to one side. When you become totally relaxed, your tongue will relax backward and cover your windpipe if you keep your head straight in line with the rest of you.

▶ Place your arms on the floor at your sides, palms down, with elbows a little bent. Flexed joints are more relaxed.

▶ Place your legs apart (not crossed or in contact with one another). As the legs relax, your feet will tend to roll outward.

▶ If you relax best with your eyes open, keep them open. If you relax best with your eyes closed, close them. If you keep them open, focus continuously on one object only.

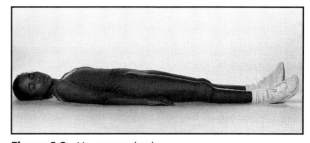

Figure 9.3. Lie on your back.

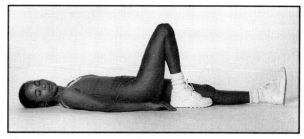

Figure 9.4. Raise one knee to relieve the arched-back feeling.

Step 2: Deep Breathing

▶ Take a deep breath and hold it in your lungs. Focus on the stretched tight feeling you get in your chest by holding in the oxygen.

▶ Now very slowly and purposefully, breathe out (through puckered lips), a long, steady exhale. Create an image in your mind to lengthen the exhale. For example, see yourself blowing the fuzzy seeds off of a dandelion that has gone to seed or blowing a long steady note on a flute.

▶ Repeat this inhale holding it, followed with another slow, steady, long exhale. Determine during this inhalation and exhalation that these next few minutes belong only to you. Do not share them with anybody or anything. Whatever problems, worries, or cares you have, including whatever it is you are going to do next in your day, briefly think what they are and list them all, by writing them on a mental chalkboard in your mind. Then, again mentally, take out a big chalk eraser and wipe each one off, one at a time, so that you are looking at an entirely blank chalkboard in your mind. Verbalize a thought to yourself like, "This is my time now (problem), and you are just going to have to wait." And then forget it during your relaxation technique!

▶ Now follow your breathing cycle, whether it is fast, slow, regular, or irregular. Just mentally tune in and follow each inhale and each exhale. Picture yourself on an elevator, and each exhale is a ride down one more floor; each inhale is the brief pause for the floor stop, door opening and closing. Or, imagine that your mind is on a slow roller coaster ride of up and down, up and down.

▶ As you begin to relax, you will experience that the exhalation (breathing out) becomes longer and longer. Don't interfere with your inhalation and exhalation — just ride with it and experience this longer ride out. This begins true relaxation.

▶ At various times during the entire body scanning relaxation technique, you will have to mentally tune back in to your breathing technique, for mastering this "elevator ride" is the central focus of your relaxation.

Step 3: Tuning In

▶ Start at the top of your head, travel down to the tips of your toes, and return to your mid-section.

▶ On the top of your head, mentally feel the "part" of your hair. Make it wide by relaxing your scalp.

▶ Mentally envision your ears. Drop all tension in your ears. If you are wearing earrings, mentally feel them on your earlobes.

▶ Tune in to your forehead. Is it tense and full of wrinkles? Make it flat, and wide with no wrinkles; picture it smooth and shiny.

▶ What is the space between your eyebrows doing? Is it grooved and full of wrinkles? Relax. Make a wide space between your eyebrows. This is one of the telltale locations of human stress. A person who is highly stressed seems to permanently keep the space between the eyebrows tensed (contracted, wrinkled). Calm, serene people stand out by having this small space wide, relaxed, and untensed.

▶ Relax your eyebrows as if heavy weights were pulling down the ends. This will also relax your temple area.

▶ There is a hinge joint near your ear hole that is used to open and close your lower jaw. Relax that mandible joint by dropping your lower jaw. It will make your lips part. Relax your chin.

▶ When you relax your jaw, mentally feel your teeth and tongue. When some people try to practice total relaxation, they tightly press (tense) their tongue to the roof of their mouths. Also, many people grit or grind their teeth at night — an audible sign of tension in the area.

▶ Relax your throat by thinking of the feeling you get with the second stage of swallowing. Persons who sing or play wind instruments have been trained in this technique to relax the area so that the best sounds will come out of a relaxed vocal mechanism.

▶ Drop your shoulders and chest so that there is a wide space between your ears and shoulders. This is an area that we unconsciously tense throughout the day, unnecessarily. Whether we drive a car or walk in miserable weather, we tense the shoulders up near our ears and encourage neckaches and headaches. When you think about it next time, untense this group if you don't actually need to be holding it in a tensed manner.

▶ Allow the weight of your chest to sink through to the floor. Think: heavy chest.

▶ Drop all tension from your upper arms, elbows, lower arms, and hands until you can just feel your fingertips pulsating on the floor. A tingling feeling may be felt in your fingertips.

▶ Relax your buttocks. This will hold the key in untensing the lower half of your body.

▶ Relax your kneecaps. This joint connects your upper and lower leg, and many times we tense our knee area when we attempt to relax other body parts. When you relax the knees, the upper legs will relax, and the heavy weight of your legs will begin to drop to the floor. Likewise, the lower legs respond almost automatically, with the feet then rolling outward.

▶ Mentally feel what your toes are doing in your shoes. Are they tensed and curled under? If so, relax them.

▶ And now, return to the most difficult place to relax — the stomach and intestinal area. Focus your mind on the navel area and picture a wide, flat, picturesque pond. Envision a small pebble being tossed into the very center, with a soft, rippling effect occurring. Each ripple is a wave of relaxation. Feel the weight of your navel area sinking through, past your spine, onto the floor below you.

▶ Now return back to your breathing cycle, and follow it several times. Remember to focus totally on the long, slow exhale.

▶ Now just **rest** a few moments and enjoy the totally untensed feeling your are experiencing.

Step 4: Heart Rate Monitoring and Stretch

▶ In this lying down position, feel for your pulse. Mentally picture and feel your heart beating. Actively try to slow it down with your mind — cue it to beat slower.

▶ Count your pulse for fifteen seconds and multiply by four for a minute heart rate count. How does this compare with your resting heart rate count after 6-8 hours of sleep? Isn't it phenomenal what three minutes of relaxation can do for your body's recovery from exercise or daily stress?

▶ You can now leave feeling totally renewed, refreshed, and in control of what remains of the rest of the day!

▶ Before you get up, sit up slowly and stretch your arms, legs, chest, back, etc. so that you become alert immediately. You must do this fifteen-second stretch or you'll find yourself yawning for an hour afterward! Of course, if this relaxation procedure is practiced before going to bed, omit this stretch.

❷ The Control Panel With One Large Dial

Throughout this *Aerobics* text, a control panel and dial visual model is used because it has been found to be the easiest to visualize and integrate into a fitness program involving change. It was used earlier for ratings of perceived exertion, it is used now for rating levels of tension and relaxation you feel within the

body, and it will be used again in Chapter 10 when developing a weight management program. Chart 19 in the Appendix entitled, "The Control Panel With One Large Dial" is provided to use in conjunction with this technique.

First, give a concrete label to each number on the control panel from 0-10, as to what that level of relaxation/tension represents to you. Maybe 0 represents totally relaxed inner peace or lying on a warm beach, 5 represents balance and peak performances, and 10 means blown away and totally out of control or experiencing death, disease, or divorce. You write entries that each number represents to you. Then, give today's best/worst moments a number; or recall your inventory resources, and list some of them on the chart where they're appropriate. Now that you have the idea of quantifying stress, visualize this second guided imagery technique.

▶ Visualize yourself in a safe place that represents relaxation to you, like perhaps your bedroom. Envision yourself there, seated in front of a control panel, which has one large dial.[4] Continue to hold onto that image in your mind's eye for the duration of the technique, and soon you will feel as if you were actually there.

▶ This large dial can be turned to any setting from 0 to 10, which represents all the various levels of relaxation and tension which you are able to experience. 0 represents all of the relaxation that's possible for you to feel, and 10 represents as much tension as you are able to experience at one time.

▶ Begin now to look very closely at this dial that directly monitors and controls the level of tension in your body. What is the reading on the dial at this moment (from zero to ten)?

▶ See yourself reaching over to turn it down. See yourself turning that dial down, v-e-r-y s-l-o-w-l-y, a little bit at a time. Feel your body relaxing more and more as you turn it down.

▶ Feel the tension in your body lessening more and more, as you turn the dial all the way down. Turn the dial all the way down to zero, as all of the tension in your body just ebbs away. Your entire body is just as relaxed as it possibly can be. All of your previous tension is replaced now with peaceful feelings of total relaxation and a centered calmness prevails.

▶ Currents of gentle tranquillity soothes every muscle, every nerve, every fiber of your being.

▶ From now on, you will be able to relax, just like this, whenever you choose, merely by sitting or lying down, closing your eyes for a few moments, and visualizing yourself turning down the dial on this control panel.

▶ You'll be able to sleep better at night, awakening more refreshed; work more efficiently without being bugged by people or situations during the day; feel rejuvenated to perform your very best when you need to; and enjoy your leisure-time activities to the fullest. Your unlimited potential awaits you in every single aspect of your life.

▶ Whether it be rest, work, or leisure, every aspect of your life will be considerably improved and enriched by your new ability to relax whenever you choose.

▶ The more you practice this new ability, the more easily and the more deeply you'll be able to relax, and the longer these feelings of relaxation will remain with you.

▶ Return now, to the moment in your day, and the location where you were, prior to your relaxation. Open your eyes and enjoy a fresh, new beginning.

3 Natural Highs

Here are experiences that most likely made you feel good in the past. Relax, close your eyes, and take a long moment to remember the best time you ever had, experiencing each one of these.

Now, create a list of your personalized natural highs from your list of resources as detailed on Chart 16 in the Appendix. First write them down and then record them on a cassette tape. Whenever your stress is out-of-control, regain balance by listening to your own natural highs.

SUMMARY

Life is a journey of many steps. We desire the pleasure that balance gives to us. We attempt to find ways to manage when imbalance (stress) enters the scene. A most enjoyable means of regaining the balance we seek is through relaxation techniques, of which there are many possibilities. This chapter presented the popular form of relaxation techniques called guided imagery. It has focused on developing an awareness toward using our own personalized resources that we have stored within, to manage the stress of our lives, through three techniques: Total Body Scanning, The Control Panel With One Large Dial, and Natural Highs.

The blueprint for mastery has been drawn. Practice is what will permanently program the management of your stress.

NATURAL HIGHS

A fun new hobby. Swimming the last lap. Singing camp songs. A long distance call from a friend. Good grades. Water-skiing. A favorite hug. Your team winning. Listening to a friend giggle. Watching a sunset. Deciding not to watch your favorite TV show to get work done, and then finding out after you finish, that your show was delayed and you still get to watch it. Your heart beat when you see someone you like. Watching an animal take a bath in a patch of sun. Intercepting a pass. New pencils and supplies on the first day of school. Eating pizza with the works. A long, hot shower. Finishing a 10-K road race. A spider web with dew on it in the early morning sun. A great book. Reading under an electric blanket on a rainy day. Your first solo bike ride. International travel. Chili dogs. Reading before and after ads about overweight people. Intimacy. A good talk with a friend. A great idea. Snowskiing, A puppy. Enthusiastic people. Climbing trees. God. Watching the moon. Plunging your hot body into a cool pool. Zoo animals nuzzling each other. An African violet that blooms. Running in the fall. Relaxing to Saturday morning cartoons. Making somebody laugh. Surfing. Walking on the beach. Decorating a Christmas tree. Playing the piano. Sailing. Fixing something that's been broken. Writing something exactly the way it has to be written to say what it has to say. A job well done. Creativity. Watching your favorite hockey team win in OT. Slumber parties. Meditation. Liking your parents. Liking your children. The quiet after a snowfall. Riding down the street in a sports car switching gears. Old college friends. Singing in the shower. Cooking somebody their favorite meal. Really observing things. A letter from a friend. Seeing a rainbow after a shower. Being appreciated. Needlework. Losing fat weight. Being noticed by somebody you've been noticing. A warm inviting smile from a stranger. Success stories. Dancing. Finishing a term paper. The first week of college. The last week of college. The day the yearbook came out. Uncontrollable laughter. Recognizing the truth in something you read. Hearing somebody say, "I love you." Holding hands. Clean hair. Stopping smoking. Stopping drugs. The first spring flower. Loving yourself. Breakfast in bed. Winks. A compassionate touch...[5]

Chapter 10

Strategies: Eating For Fitness, Weight Management, and Goal Setting

CHOICES

"Choose what is best; habit will soon render it agreeable and easy." Ancient philosopher Pythagoras stated this principle of making choices many years ago and it hasn't really changed today. Better or best choices are available for you to make. Become informed as to what is best, then choose well repeatedly. The actions you take will become blueprinted and your mindset will be established for making fitness choices. Take a look now at better or best choices to make in regards to:

▶ proper eating;

▶ managing your weight; and

▶ setting total-program goals for yourself.
Fitness is a *choice*.

Eating For Fitness Is A Choice

Your body has two basic types of nutrient needs:

▶ Foods that satisfy your energy needs.

▶ Foods that provide the growth, repair, and regulation-of-body-processes needs.

Nutrients are chemical substances that your body absorbs from food during digestion. Over 40 nutrients are known to be needed by your body through your diet. *Diet* here means total intake of food and drink. Essential nutrients are those that your body cannot make or is unable to make in adequate amounts. These nutrients must be obtained from what you eat and drink. If they are not properly provided through your diet your body cannot perform well, mentally or physically.

This is where your choice comes in. You may know what the better choices of foods are, called *nutrient dense* foods[1], but if you don't eat the best choices available to you, you really don't know good nutrition at all. Good health, optimum fitness, or good nutrition is not just knowing what is best, but choosing it 80 to 90 percent of the time.[2]

Best Choices For A Balanced Diet

A well-balanced diet is one that contains the following six basic nutrients. Proper amounts of each are established according to your age, gender, activity level, and state of wellness:

▶ Carbohydrates

▶ Fats

▶ Proteins

▶ Vitamins

▶ Minerals

▶ Water

And, note the following:

▶ All persons need the same nutrients all their lives but in varying amounts.

▶ Larger amounts are needed for growth than for maintaining the body.

▶ Pre-adolescent children need smaller amounts of food/nutrients than adults, although they need the same ones.

▶ Boys and men need and use more nutrients and energy than girls and women.

► The only exception to the aforementioned is the need for iron. Women of child-bearing age need more iron than other people.

► Active people require more nutrients that provide energy than inactive people.

► People recovering from illness need more nutrients than when in good health.[3]

These nutrients can be supplied by eating from the four food groups as illustrated in the pamphlet "Guide to Good Eating" published by the National Dairy Council,[4] and shown in Figures 10.1–10.4. It is not always possible to intake all of the essential nutrients every twenty-four hours. What *is* important is that over a span of several days and weeks, there is a continual selection from the four groups to meet nutrient needs.

Nutrient Density

It is best to consider the unique concept of nutrient density when making these selections, however. Following the figures of each food group shown here, foods have been listed according to *nutrient density* — that is, *the amount of nutrition per calorie each food provides.* To get the most nutrition for the least calories, choose foods from the four star groups, which are even ranked within each starred group and listed in descending order of nutrients per calorie.[5] Nutrient Density information is reprinted with permission from Nutrition Education Services, Oregon Dairy Council. The categories are:

► 4 stars — most nutrition per calorie

► 3 stars — next to most nutrition per calorie

► 2 stars — next to least nutrition per calorie

► 1 star — least nutrition per calorie.[6]

Knowing this ranking will help you to make better choices consistently when a variety is available from which to select. If you make the better or best choices most of the time, your body will be fueled and ready to perform optimally, both physically and mentally.

A final point to be made in regards to food choices is that if you know little about human physiology (how your vital processes work), it's best not to resort to chance or just any source for nutritional guidelines. There is an abundance of excellent scientifically-based, yet easy to read, literature available that has been researched with controls and explains what is entailed in the balancing of these six needed basic nutrients. The best choice regarding nutritional guidelines and information to follow is to select those developed by the well-established medical and fitness professionals, rather than those from your favorite movie and television stars or the supermarket trade magazines.

THE FOUR FOOD GROUPS
Milk Group

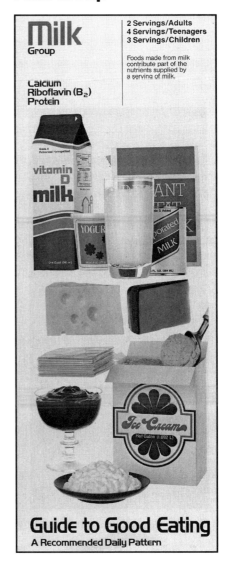

Figure 10.1.

Rating:	Food Choices in Ranked Order:	Serving:
****	nonfat plain yogurt,	
	nonfat milk,	1 cup (8 oz.);
	lowfat cheese,	1 ounce (cheese)
	buttermilk, lowfat plain	
	yogurt, 1%-2% milk	1 cup (8 oz.)
***	regular fat cheese,	
	ricotta cheese,	1 ounce
	whole milk, kefir, lowfat	
	yogurt w/fruit,	1 cup
	lowfat chocolate milk,	
	nonfat frozen yogurt	1 cup
**	pudding, custard	1 cup
	lowfat frozen yogurt,	
	ice milk	1½ cups
*	cottage cheese	2 cups
	milkshake	1½ cups
	Kissle	1 cup
	ice cream	1½ cups

Note: Nutrient density figured for **calcium**.

The Milk Group is the only group in which the serving sizes change in reference to your age. Adults need two servings except pregnant or lactating women, who need four servings; growing, pre-adolescent children need three servings; and teen-agers need four servings. Calcium, riboflavin (vitamin B_2), and protein are the key nutrients that are needed to build the basic structure and strength of bones and teeth, assist in the production of energy needs, and help in the growth and maintenance of every living cell.

If you are not an avid milk fan, you can eat any of the foods in the milk group and it will supply the cal-cium, riboflavin, and protein that you need. Again, for the best nutrition per calorie, foods are listed and starred.

Rating:	Food Choices in Ranked Order:	Serving:
****	lean cuts of: beef, veal, fish, pork, lamb, poultry, (visible fat removed);	2-3 ounces, cooked
	eggs	2
***	regular and higher fat cuts of: beef, fish, pork, lamb, poultry, (visible fat **not** removed);	2-3 ounces cooked
	tofu	7 ounces
	dried beans, peas, lentils	1 cup cooked
**	nuts and seeds	½ cup
*	peanut butter	4 Tblsp.
	hot dog, luncheon meats, sausage	2-3 ounces

Note: Nutrient density figured for **iron** and **protein**.

Meat Group

This group is called the "meat group," but there are also plant foods that, when eaten together, supply the needed protein, niacin, iron, and thiamine and are then considered an alternative choice to eating meat.

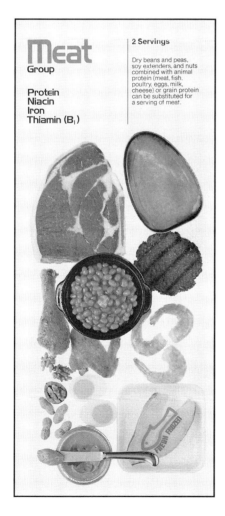

Figure 10.2.

Some of the plant foods that can be combined so that their proteins complement each other (i.e., allow the amino acids to combine to form balanced pro-tein) are: dried beans and whole wheat, dried beans and corn or rice, or peanuts and wheat.[7]

All persons need two servings per day of the meat group (except pregnant women, who need three servings per day). One serving is equal to two ounces of cooked lean meat, fish, or poultry, or the protein equivalent. Visually, a 2 ounce portion is equal in size to the palm of an average hand, and the width of the little finger.

Count cheeses as servings of meat or milk, but not simultaneously.[8] Remember to strip all excess fat off any meat that you eat. Remove the skin from poultry, and eat only the meat. You will thus eliminate un-necessary calories.

Fruit and Vegetable Group

This group provides vitamins A and C, which are actually catalysts or action starters. The most impor-tant functions of these vitamins include:

▶ Formation and maintenance of skin and body linings.

▶ Cementing substances to promote strength in cells and hasten healing of injuries.

▶ Functions in all visual processes.

▶ Aids in the use of iron.

These are all functions that you want to enjoy, so be sure not to slight this group.

All persons need four servings per day. One serving is:

▶ Medium size whole fruit or vegetable

▶ 1 cup raw

► 1/2 cup cooked
► 1/2-3/4 cup juice
► 1/4 cup dried fruit

Sources of Vitamin A

Orange and green. Remembering two simple colors will help you remember that foods of these colors will provide Vitamin A. It is recommended that dark green, leafy, or orange vegetables and fruits be eaten at least every other day (such as carrots, sweet potatoes, or greens). Because vitamin A is stored in the fat tissue of the body, an overdose through supplementation in pill form can be fatal. (The same is true for the other fat-soluble vitamins: D, E, and K.)

Sources of Vitamin C

Fruits and vegetables such as broccoli, oranges, grapefruits, or strawberries are recommended daily for supplying the needed catalyst, vitamin C. This vitamin is water-soluble, which means that if too much is intaken, the extra is excreted through the urine. If you decide to take vitamin C supplement pills in massive doses, your body reacts by increasing the level it needs. If you then suddenly stop taking vitamin C supplements, your body reacts as if it were deficient! So supplementation is costly and unnecessary for well persons who eat properly.

Rating:	Food Choices in Ranked Order:
****	spinach, chard, broccoli, cantaloupe, tomatoes, brussels sprouts, asparagus, kale, green peppers, winter squash, romaine lettuce
***	vegetable juice, zucchini, green beans, oranges, cabbage, cauliflower, sweet potatoes, apricots, cucumbers, orange juice, carrots, grapefruit, celery
**	artichokes, strawberries, peas, corn, bananas, potatoes, beets, peaches, iceberg lettuce, sprouts, mushrooms, pears, avocados, pineapple juice
*	apples, raisins, grapes, canned fruit, dried fruit, french fries

Note: Nutrient density figured for **folic acid**, **Vitamins A** and **C**.

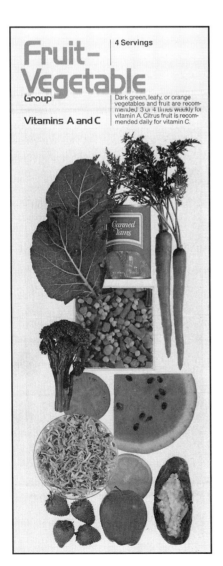

Figure 10.3.

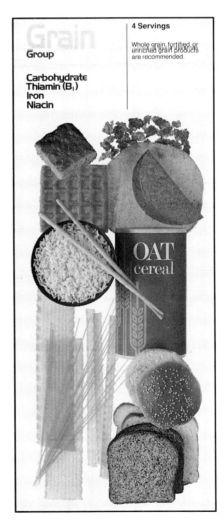

Figure 10.4.

Grain Group (Whole, Fortified, Enriched)

Although this group assists with the growth and maintenance of cells and with the elimination process (fiber provides bulk to your waste for easy removal), the major function is to provide *energy*. Your number one daily need is energy so that you are able to perform every single daily function from sleeping to aerobics.

Four servings per day is the minimum amount required by all groups. Remember, if you do not: use this carbohydrate food for the expenditure of energy, use it for growth and repair, or eliminate it, you wear it as body fat — future energy. It's like constantly carrying around extra gasoline for your car.

A minimum amount of four servings is suggested as a daily intake. Look again to see exactly how much a serving is. It is, again, not all you consume or serve yourself at one time, but a measured amount of food. If you wish to lose fat weight, watch the amount of additional energy food that you intake. If, however, you are an active person — a varsity or endurance athlete — you will *want* to provide an abundance of this energy food.

Rating:	Food Choices in Ranked Order:	Serving:
****	bran (1/3 cup) and whole grain (1 cup) cereals,	1/3-1 cup ready-to-eat or 1/2 cup cooked;
	whole wheat breads and rolls,	1 slice or 1/2 bun;
	whole grain crackers,	4
	corn tortillas	1
***	pasta/noodles, brown rice,	1/2 cup
	enriched breads and rolls,	1 slice or 1/2 bun;
	cornbread	2" square
**	flour tortilla	1
	bagel	1/2
	plain muffin	1
	graham and saltine crackers	4
	pancakes	1
	other cereals	1 cup
	granola type cereal	1/3 cup
	pita bread	1/2 pocket
*	breadsticks (3), English muffin (1/2), enriched rice (1/2 cup cooked), biscuit (1), stuffing (1/2 cup cooked), croissant (1/2).	

Note: Nutrient density figured for **fiber**.

Combination Foods

These items comprise more than one food group. They count as servings (or partial servings) from the groups from which they were made.

Some of the food choices are: burritos, casseroles, chef salad, hamburgers, lasagna, macaroni and cheese, pizza, soup, stew, tacos.

Extras/Others/"Sometimes" Foods

There is no recommended number of servings for the foods classified as extras. These food choices provide little or no nutrition and are often very high in sugar, salt, fat and calories. These foods are classified as Extras: alcoholic beverages, bacon, bouillon, butter, cakes, candy, coffee, cookies, condiments, cream, cream cheese, doughnuts, fruit flavored drinks, gelatin dessert, gravy, honey, jam, jelly, margarine, mayonnaise, non-dairy creamer, olives, onion rings, pickles, pies, popcorn, potato chips, pretzels, salad dressings, sauces, seasonings, sherbet, soft drinks, sour cream, sugar, tea, tortilla chips, vegetable oils.[9]

MONITORING FOOD AND BEVERAGE INTAKE

Do you eat a wide variety of foods in moderation from the Four Food Groups? Use Chart 18 located in the Appendix entitled, "My Daily Consumption" to discover what your eating plan is. Start by thinking about what you had to eat today and record the foods you ate after the appropriate food group.

For a combination food, think about what foods went into it and list those foods under the appropriate food group. For example, the cheese on a pizza would be recorded in the milk group, the tomatoes

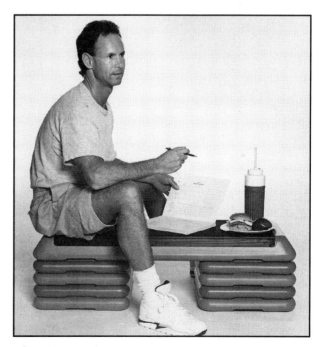

Figure 10.5.

and any other vegetables should be recorded in the fruit-vegetable group, and the crust is recorded in the grain group. The ingredients in a combination food may not always count as a full serving from the food group. Remember to think in terms of quantity of servings, along with the nutrient category it's listed under.

Continue monitoring your intake for one week. How does it measure up to the standards established for a balanced diet with special attention on selecting nutrient dense foods? If your diet lacks foods from one of the food groups, variety, or moderation, you may not be getting all the nutrients and energy you need. It's easy to improve your diet if you take it one step at a time.

Start by choosing one challenge to work on, come up with a solution, and spend one week trying to correct it. After it's mastered, choose a second eating challenge that needs attention, and continue until you have your diet well-managed.

Nutrition and the Athlete

Guidelines

The proper food intake of the athlete is the starting point for training or conditioning. The food groups already presented form the *foundation* of the diet recommended for young athletes. This plan serves as the nucleus for meals both in and out of athletic seasons. There is a vast leeway in the choice of the foods within each of the food groups. Major deviations for athletes from these food groups should rarely be necessary. Basic nutritional needs of athletes and nonathletes do not differ except for caloric needs.[10]

Total caloric needs vary with individual metabolism and physical activity. An intake of 2000 calories each day should be the bare minimum allowed for an athlete involved in a vigorous training program. The amount of calories expended by a young male athlete in serious training may range as high as 4000-6000 calories per day. Remember, however, calorie intake that exceeds expenditure for basal body functions, for physical activity, and for growth of lean body mass, will form body fat!

The Pre-Game Diet

A pre-game meal should:
▶ Support blood sugar levels to avoid hunger sensations.
▶ Leave the stomach and upper bowel empty at the time of competition.
▶ Provide maximum hydration.
▶ Minimize stomach upset; promote maximum performance.

▶ Provide a psychological edge by including foods the athlete likes and believes will make him or her win.

1 *Carbohydrates* in the diet will support blood sugar and provide glycogen stores to maintain these levels. Glycogen is the storage form of carbohydrate and seems to be the quickest and most efficient source of energy.

Good choices of high carbohydrate foods are: apples, applesauce, bagels, baked potatoes, baking powder biscuits, bananas, boiled potatoes, bread, (white, whole wheat), cheese pizza, egg noodles, graham crackers, a hard roll, macaroni and cheese, mashed potatoes, oatmeal, an orange, orange juice, orange sherbet, pancakes (enriched), a pear, spaghetti (cooked), sponge cake, sweet potatoes, and waffles.

2 You may wonder which foods are easily digested and will leave the stomach empty for the competition. Again, carbohydrates are more rapidly digested than protein and fat. (A breakfast of

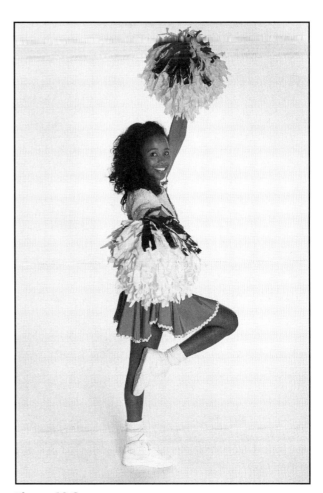

Figure 10.6.

toast and jam, cereal with low-fat milk, and fruit or juice will leave the stomach much sooner than a meal of eggs with steak, sausage, or bacon.)

3 Optimum hydration is very important to the athlete, especially to those involved in endurance events, such as long-distance swimming or running. The immediate pre-game diet should consist of 2 to 3 glasses of some beverage, with no less than eight full glasses each 24 hours.

Whole milk is not recommended because of its high fat content; caffeine should also be avoided because it may increase nervous tension and agitation before the contest. Non-carbonated fruit drinks are generally a good choice.

4 Very concentrated sources of simple sugar such as glucose tablets or undiluted honey should be avoided as they can cause gas distention and discomfort. Also, very bulky foods high in fiber or cellulose would not be a good choice before an event.

Heavily salted foods should probably be avoided on the day of competition because they can cause water retention, which decreases athletic performance.

5 The pre-game meal should be eaten from three to four hours before the contest. If you engage in a very demanding sport, a 1000-calorie meal would be ideal. A 500 calorie meal would suffice for a sport demanding lower energy.

In conclusion, athletes make special demands on their bodies and must be physically prepared to met those demands. The starting block is sound nutrition knowledge and practice. Don't sacrifice a winning excellence to an inefficient or harmful diet. Reduced strength and endurance and a poor performance would be your result.

Vegetarianism Principles

Adults can get all nutrients in adequate amounts from a carefully planned vegetarian diet. This is especially true if milk and eggs are included along with a variety of plant-source foods, including dried beans and peas, nuts, dark-green leafy vegetables, and fruits.

On the other hand, the nutritional risk of a vegetarian diet increases as more foods are excluded. If you follow vegetarianism and exclude all foods of animal origin (including milk and eggs), you will need to plan very carefully in order to obtain enough of the nutrients protein, calcium, iron, and vitamin

D. Furthermore, sufficient vitamin B_{12}, which is found only in animal-source foods, may be a problem. A vitamin B_{12} pill or soy milk fortified with B_{12} should be taken.

For most people, a vegetarian diet which includes milk and eggs is adequate, provided it is planned carefully. However, if you are growing or have a digestive or other health problem, you should get professional help from a dietitian or doctor to be sure your vegetarian diet meets your needs.

Vegetarianism Words & Phrases

▶ **Brewer's and Torula Yeast** — A good source of several vitamins; it also contains some protein and minerals. It does not have rising properties like baking yeast.

▶ **Complete Protein** — A protein that contains all eight of the essential amino acids. Meats, milk products, and eggs are all complete proteins. Mixing together vegetables and grain proteins can also make a complete protein.

▶ **Legumes** — The seed of a pod-bearing plant, including peas, beans, soybeans, lentils, and peanuts. Legumes are good sources of protein.

▶ **Meat Analog** — A formulated plant-protein food simulating meat or meat products.

▶ **Soy Milk** — The liquid which remains after soaking and straining soybeans. Treatment with heat plus fortification with vitamin B_{12} makes soy milk a protein-rich beverage which can be used like cow's milk.

▶ **Taboule** — A Middle Eastern bean and wheat salad which provides complete protein.

▶ **Tofu** — A curd or cheese made from fresh soybeans. Originating in Asia, tofu is a good source of protein and can be used in salads, soups, sauces, vegetable casseroles, egg dishes, and even desserts.

▶ **Triticale** — A grain hybrid between wheat and rye that has a richer protein content than wheat. Triticale flour has different baking qualities than wheat flour.[11]

Eating Out Tips
Fast Foods:

▶ In fast food restaurants, select the smallest burger.

▶ Choose milk instead of a milkshake.

▶ Try taking an apple along and eat it instead of fries.

▶ Use ketchup or mustard and ask to hold the mayonnaise or tartar sauce. (This is a good idea for home, too.)

▶ Extra crispy fried chicken has more calories and fat than regular fried chicken.

▶ A plain roast beef sandwich has less fat than a fried chicken or fish sandwich.

▶ Fast food breakfasts tend to be high in fat and calories. Choose cereal with milk, fruit or juice, plain toast, English muffin, fruit muffin, or bagle. Plain pancakes are lower in fat than breakfast sandwiches. Don't add butter or margarine and go lightly on the syrup.

▶ Salad bars are a healthy option. Choose lettuce or other greens, and stick with the plain fresh fruits and vegetables. Watch mayonnaise-based items such as potato salad or macaroni salad. Watch items such as bacon bits and salad dressing. Use sparingly!

▶ Soft ice cream has the lowest calories and fat of most desserts generally available on fast-food menus. A plain soft ice cream cone has around 190 calories and 5 grams of fat. Cookies and pies have about 100 calories more, and a much higher percentage of their calories come from fat.

Restaurant Dining:

▶ Look for foods that are steamed, poached, broiled or fresh rather than fried, creamed, crispy, breaded or basted.

▶ When ordering, ask that the sauce be left off your sandwich or entree and salad dressing be served on the side.

▶ Choose salads that are served fresh or plain rather than pre-mixed with mayonnaise, oil or creamy dressings.

▶ Choose whole grain bread or rolls.

▶ Try fresh fruit, angel food cake, lowfat frozen yogurt or fruit ices for dessert.

▶ Choose baked potatoes in place of french fries or potatoes in sauce. Go easy on sour cream, butter, margarine, and other high fat additions sparingly.

▶ Watch the portion size of your main dish. Most restaurant entrees give you more than you need. Don't hesitate to ask for a doggie bag.[12]

Eating In — Convenience Tips

Frozen dinners have become an integral part of our diet. There's a very simple reason for the ever-increasing popularity of frozen entrees. They are very convenient! The only problem as far as today's health-conscious consumers are concerned is trying to figure out which ones fit easily into a nutritious diet.

Tufts University has published a list of 108 frozen dinners[13] that can be made effortlessly into your main meal mainstays if you are choosing to eat to stay healthy as well as remain or become trim. These dinners have been commercially marketed to those people who want to limit their intake of fat, calories, and sodium, while including in their diets essential vitamins and minerals. You can enjoy these frozen dishes without wondering whether they have a place in your healthful eating plan.

The strict standards used to develop this list could not cover every single nutrient; some meals will be low in certain vitamins and minerals. To compensate for this, they have also developed a very comprehensive list of 50 easy-to-put-together, 100-200 calorie side dishes. Any one of these will add the missing amounts of vitamin A and C, along with some fiber. Many of the dinners lack the fiber that will help you leave the table feeling full because they contain bulk. Send for this information[14] if your meals are based on the convenience frozen dinners provide.

Water: Bottled Varieties

This key nutrient has been given a variety of names according to the components it contains. Bottled water companies that are members of the International Bottled Water Association are inspected yearly, so look for their labels which carry the important "NSF" certification.[15]

Be aware that 25 percent of bottled waters are little more than packaged tap water. There is nothing illegal about a company using water from the source of a public supply and selling it in plastic containers or bottles.[16] Also note that bottled water may not contain the right amount of fluoride to fight cavities.

The following are six varieties of bottled water and their specific characteristics:

Natural water is water that is not derived from a municipal system or public supply and has not been modified by the addition or deletion of any minerals.

Spring water flows out of the earth on its own at a particular spot and is bottled at or near its source. It is unmodified by the addition or deletion of minerals if its bottler is a member of the International Bottled Water Association.

Purified water, also known as distilled (vaporized and recondensed) water, is completely demineralized. It has what is often called a flat taste that many people consider objectionable.

Mineral water, technically speaking, is any water that is not distilled, but to the International Bottled Water Association, it's water that "contains not less than 500 parts per million total dissolved solids." The more solids, or minerals, the stronger the water's taste.

Club soda is water that has been artifically carbonated (with carbon dioxide) and contains added salts and minerals.

Seltzer is also injected with carbon dioxide but has no added salts.[17]

Dietary Guidelines for Americans

Food alone cannot make you healthy. But good eating habits based on moderation and variety can help keep you healthy and even improve your health. The following guidelines suggested for most Americans were developed by the U.S. Department of Agriculture, U.S. Department of Health and Human Services, and are printed in more complete detail in the pamphlet, "Nutrition and Your Health: Dietary Guidelines for Americans."[18] In brief, it is suggested that Americans need to pay more attention to the following.

1 *Eat a variety of foods.* No single food item supplies all the essential nutrients in the amounts you need. The greater the variety, the less likely you are to develop either a deficiency or an excess of any single nutrient.

2 *Maintain healthy weight.* If you are too fat or too thin, your chances of developing health problems are increased (i.e., high blood pressure, diabetes, heart disease, certain cancers, etc.). There is no one plan for maintaining healthy weight. If your concern is to lose fat weight, try increasing your physical activity, eating less fat and fatty foods, eating less sugar and sweets, and avoiding too much alcohol.

3 *Choose a diet low in fat, saturated fat, and cholesterol.* If you have a high blood cholesterol level, you have a greater chance of having a heart attack. Populations like ours with diets high in saturated fats and cholesterol tend to have high blood cholesterol levels.

There is controversy about what recommendations are appropriate for healthy Americans. But for the U.S. population as a whole, a reduction in our current intake of total fat, saturated fat, and cholesterol is sensible.

▶ Choose lean meats, fish, poultry, dry beans, and peas as your protein sources.

▶ Moderate your use of eggs and organ meats (such as liver).

▶ Limit your intake of butter, cream hydrogenated margarines, shortenings, and coconut oil, and foods made from such products.

▶ Trim excess fat off meats.

▶ Broil, bake, or boil rather than fry.

▶ Read labels carefully to determine amounts and types of fat contained in foods.

Important dietary goals to remember:

▶ Cholesterol — consume 300 mg/day or less.

▶ Fat — should be 30% of daily calories or less.

When reading labels, to determine the percentage of calories in a product that come from fat:

▶ Remember that one gram of fat equals 9 calories.

▶ Multiply the grams of fat in a serving times 9. The result equals the number of calories from fat in a serving.

▶ Divide the fat calories by the total calories in a serving to determine the percent. For example, if a chili label reads 1 cup serving = 200 calories/Fat 10 gm/Carbohydrate 5 gm/Sodium 980 mg.: There are 10 grams of fat in 1 cup of chili. 10 grams of fat × 9 calories = 90 calories from fat in 1 cup. 90 ÷ 200 = 45% of the calories in 1 cup of chili come from fat![19]

4 *Choose a diet with plenty of vegetables, fruits, and grain products.* The major sources of energy in the average U.S. diet are carbohydrates and fats. Carbohydrates have an advantage over fats: They contain less than half the number of calories per ounce than fats.

Complex carbohydrate foods are better than simple carbohydrates. Simple carbohydrates (sugars) provide calories for energy but little else in the way of nutrients. Complex carbohydrates (beans, nuts, fruits, whole grain breads) contain many essential nutrients plus calories for energy.

Increasing your consumption of certain complex carbohydrates can also help increase dietary fiber, which tends to reduce the symptoms of chronic constipation, diverticulosis, and some types of irritable bowel. There is also concern that diets low in fiber content might also increase the risk of developing cancer of the colon. Eating fruits, vegetables, and whole grain breads and cereals will provide adequate fiber in the diet.

5 *Use sugars only in moderation.* The major hazard from eating too much sugar is tooth decay. The risk increases:

▶ The more frequently you eat sugar and sweets, especially between meals.

▶ If you eat foods that stick to the teeth (sticky candy, dates, daylong use of soft drinks).

To avoid excess sugar:

▶ Use less of all sugars (white, brown, raw, honey, and syrups).

▶ Select fresh fruit or fruit canned without heavy syrup.

▶ Read food labels for sugar included — sucrose, glucose, maltose, dextrose, lactose, fructose, or syrup. If it's one of the first ingredients, a lot of sugar is inside.

To determine how many teaspoons of sugar a product contains:

▶ Remember that there are 5 grams of sugar in 1 teaspoon.

▶ Therefore, divide the grams in a serving by 5. For example, if a cereal box label reads 1 cup serving = 140 calories/carbohydrates> Starch 10 gm/ sucrose 15 grams/fiber 1 gm.: There are 15 grams of sucrose in 1 cup of cereal. 15 grams of sucrose ÷ 5 = 3 teaspoons of simple sugar in 1 cup of cereal! Products are "healthier" when sucrose (simple sugar) amounts are kept low.[20]

6 *Use salt and sodium only in moderation.* The major hazard of excessive sodium is how it affects your blood pressure. In populations where high-sodium intake is common, high blood pressure is likewise common. In populations where low-sodium intake occurs, high blood pressure is rare. Establish preventative measures early, such as:

▶ Eliminate all salt use at the table.

▶ Cook with no or very little salt.

▶ Select foods that are low in sodium content.

The dietary goal for sodium intake is approximately 2000-3000 mg/day. Be informed of the following foods containing a relatively high sodium content:

Food	Serving Size	Mg/Sodium Content
antacid (in water)	1 dose	564 mg.
canned corn	1 cup	384
cottage cheese	4 ounces	457
dill pickle	1	928
ham	3 ounces	1114
salt	1 tsp.	1938
tomato sauce	1 cup	1498

7

If you drink alcohol, do so in moderation. Alcoholic beverages tend to be high in calories and low in other nutrients. Heavy drinkers may lose their appetites for foods that contain essential nutrients. Vitamin and mineral deficiencies occur commonly in heavy drinkers:

▶ Because of poor nutrient intake.

▶ Because alcohol alters absorption and use of some essential nutrients.

It has been said that education leads to *moderation* in all areas of life. One or two drinks daily appear to cause no harm in adults. However, even moderate drinkers need to remember that alcohol is a high-calorie, low-nutrient food, and if you wish to achieve or maintain ideal weight, the intake must be well monitored.

WHAT IS MODERATE DRINKING?

Women: No more than 1 drink a day
Men: No more than 2 drinks a day.

Count as a drink:

▶ 12 ounces of regular beer

▶ 5 ounces of wine

▶ 1 ½ ounces of distilled spirits (80 proof)[21]

WEIGHT MANAGEMENT

When asked why they are taking a fitness course, most persons will respond, "to improve my physique by toning muscles and losing weight." A simple yet concrete goal. We seem to readily admit to the fact that a primary goal is to *appear* healthy and slim — to either ourselves or to others.

Why do individuals today desire this goal? It's because we can directly see when our body looks nice, lean, and toned; likewise, we can directly see when it looks out of shape, flabby, and full of fat deposits. When it comes to improvement, many individuals will therefore initially focus on this concrete form of their understanding of "fitness" or "being in shape" that they can directly see.

Your outer appearance is not, however, the entire, or even major focus, of a quality fitness program. It was mentioned earlier that you can live without well-toned muscles or a trim figure, but you can't live long without a good strong heart and lungs. It is difficult for many people to have life-sustaining goals, such as heart and lung fitness, uppermost in mind, because you just can't see your heart, lungs, or blood vessels. Therefore, acknowledging and understanding the accompanying facets and the admitted personal priorities that people bring to a fitness program is indeed necessary. Looking attractive and feeling good about and accepting your appearance are important ancillary goals to have and understand. Since you can directly and concretely see and experience this quality, and admit to this being a top priority anyway, let's next consider weight management.

Weight Management

Weight management equals controlling the amount of body fat that you carry in relation to the amount of lean you have. The principles of weight management include all of the following: *weight maintenance* (keeping the same ratio of fat to amount of lean you carry), *weight gain* (almost always in terms of lean weight gain, not fat weight gain), and *weight loss* (always in terms of loss of body fat).

Weight Maintenance

This refers to the fact that:

▶ Your current composition of fat to lean is ideal for your best cardiorespiratory health.

▶ You are pleased with how you look. You have enough strength to function well in your daily life of work and recreation, to whatever extreme that may encompass. To remain at this constant weight, your energy must be in balance:

calories in = calories out
eating = expenditure; exercise

Since a decline in calories out occurs with aging (your metabolism slows down and you are less active), a decline in calories in (eating less) must accompany the aging processes.

Weight Gain

This almost always refers to the gaining of lean tissue, or the thickening of muscle fiber. When you want to cosmetically look better, or to have an increased amount of strength for a sport or for daily needs, weight training is the type of activity in which to engage. Since you would be using more energy in a day than you did prior to the weight training program, you would need to "calories in" (eat) the same amount as you are newly expending (in the form of "calories out") with weight training, for maintenance. However, to *gain lean and lose extra body fat* simultaneously requires you to eat less while providing the *increased exercise* of weight training. Only if you are at ideal weight or underfat weight should you accompany this weight-gain program with an increase in caloric intake.[22]

Weight gain would then directly mean an increase in muscle mass, or the thickening of your muscle fibers. You primarily do not gain more muscle cells — you thicken what you presently have.

Weight Loss

This always refers to the purposeful losing of *fat weight* — never lean weight. Weight loss, of course, can occur to both your lean and your fat, according to how you go about losing the weight. The director of the local Better Business Bureau has stated that one of the top two frauds with which he comes in contact involves weight loss products and information. Before you spend your money on any claim, product, device, or book, call your local Better Business Bureau. However, if you understand the principles of weight loss, you will always be able to determine a product's, or program's, worth before you spend time, money, and energy on it.

Principles of Weight Loss (i.e., Fat Loss)

1 *Fat weight is the only kind of weight to lose.* When a product or program claims to "get rid of excess body fluids," beware! Body fluids are not fat! Incidentally, unnatural water retention, or edema, is a condition to be monitored and treated by a doctor, not by your self-prescribed procedures or products.

2 *If you lose water weight (fluids) by sweating during exercise, you will and should, gain it back in twenty-four hours* to maintain your body's synchronized chemical balance. The energy-producing (metabolic) processes perform best when all of the necessary components are present. So don't be misled into believing that dropping your water weight is effective weight loss. It is part of your fat-free weight and is a vital part of your continuous well-being. You can understand, then why weighing yourself after a strenuous exercise session is an inaccurate time to weigh.

3 *Fat is metabolized more readily and efficiently by performing moderate intensity exercise for a long duration of time.* If you are able to work continuously at a moderate intensity (lower end of your training zone), for over thirty minutes, you will have provided yourself with the most physiologically sound way to metabolize (burn off) that unwanted body fat.

So the key is: you need to exercise for more than thirty minutes at a time to make significant changes in the fat content of the body.

Wearing rubber suits, transparent plastic wrap around body parts, and on hot days heavy, long-sleeved sweats, nylons, or tights will tend to inhibit the free flow of sweat and will disallow it to perform its function of cooling you. When it is hot and humid, wear as little as possible when performing fitness exercises. You cannot metabolize (burn up) fat faster by increasing your body temperature by wearing more clothes!

4   *Fat will burn off your body in a general way.* You can't "spot reduce!" Spot reducing is perhaps the most prevalent misconception concerning fat weight loss and the one by which many unscrupulous people are defrauding unsuspecting overfat Americans out of millions of dollars every year.

By your genetic constitution, your body will use up its stored energy (fat) any way in which it is programmed to do so. You cannot do fifty leg lifts a day and hope to reduce the fat deposits in the area. You will shape up (thicken) the muscle fiber in the area, and toned muscles contain more of the enzymes involved in breaking down fat, but you do not burn off the fat there, or at any one particular location, necessarily. As energy is needed, it is withdrawn — first from the immediate sources — and when this is used up, it is withdrawn randomly from more permanent storage. It is then converted to an immediate usable form. Thus, you may lose weight in places you don't necessarily wish to at first, like your face, chest/breast area, etc. But with a little perseverance, you'll burn off the fat in problem areas, too.

5   *Fat weight loss is most readily accomplished through a combined program of dieting and exercising.* It is very difficult to lose fat weight by only exercising more, and not changing your eating habits (less "calories in"). And when you only diet (eat less food) and step on a scale, the weight loss is not all fat! According to the way in which you have dieted, your weight loss is approximately one-half to two-thirds (50 to 68 percent) fat loss and one-third to one-half (33 to 50 percent) lean weight loss. And if your lifestyle and habits of eating and exercising don't change, after you stop dieting and you gain back your lost weight, what you gain back is all fat. You are therefore worse off! You lost both fat and lean and regained back only fat. Over a lifetime of this "yo-yo" crash dieting, you can see how you are detrimentally changing your entire body composition.

When you diet (by eating less) and exercise (expending more calories or energy), you tend to lose approximately 100 percent fat. This is the only kind of weight that you want to lose. Exercise speeds weight loss, not only by burning calories while you're working out, but also by revitalizing your metabolism so that you continue to burn calories more readily for the next few hours.

6   *You can gain and lose weight with an endurance exercise program.* You will be burning off fat for energy and building up muscle simultaneously. So if you do not realize a change on the scale immediately, don't be disappointed.

7   *A light exercise program will tend to increase your appetite, and a strenuous exercise program will decrease your appetite.* You will especially find that after an endurance (aerobic) hour, your desire for food greatly diminishes. You will have time to carefully select or prepare what you know is good for you, rather than ravenously grab that easy, high-calorie junk food just sitting around.

8   *It is easier to eat less food than it is to exercise it off.* In most high-intensity fitness sessions, you will only burn about 300 calories. So think twice about rewarding yourself with high-calorie treats afterward if you are seriously interested in losing your extra fat weight. Instead, replenish your water loss with non-calorie, yet quite filling, ice water.

9   *There is no such thing as a constipated endurance aerobic exerciser or athlete.* Regular, rhythmic stimulation of the entire digestion and elimination processes will be one of the side benefits that you'll not necessarily talk about, but for which you will certainly be glad!

10   *The basic principle for fat weight loss is that the body's energy balance determines whether or not a person gains or loses body fat.* There simply is no easy "magic" way — just self-discipline to understand that proper weight loss is the result, if less caloric energy is taken in and more caloric energy is expended.

Weight Loss Strategies

A single problem such as being overweight may involve the need for any or all of the following: 1) better self image; 2) a naturally slender eating strategy; 3) learning effective ways to motivate and decide; 4) resolving a phobic response to childhood abuse; 5) learning better social skills; or 6) learning better coping skills.[23]

 Strategy For "Naturally Slender" Eating

One of the key differences between naturally slender people and overweight individuals is the construction of their mental images and self-talk concerning food. Overweight persons usually construct present-tense pictures and self-talk. They see, smell, hear, experience food, and state internally, "Boy, am I hungry!," and the result is that they immediately eat. They focus only on the pleasurable taste of food as they eat.

Naturally thin persons usually do not have this present-tense strategy. They create future-tense pictures, self-talk, feelings, etc. They experience how they'll feel over a period of time.[24] Those future pictures and words help them to be masters at weight management and they then can enjoy the pleasurable selections they make.

 Control Panel With One Large Dial

Chart 19 in the Appendix was used in conjunction with rating the tension and relaxation you experienced from your stressors. This same control panel can be used as an eating strategy, Chart 20.

Give each number a representation for how full you feel. Begin with the 5 representing "feeling very comfortable and full," and label in both directions from there. Here are some suggestions for labels with corresponding numbers to get you started, but remember to label the control panel the way you want to, concerning how you feel.

0-1   Starved/Famished
  2   The beginning of a meal
  3   Only half-full
  4   Not quite satisfied
  5   Feeling very comfortable and full
  6   Should have omitted extra-helping, or dessert
  7   Absolutely stuffed; ate and drank enough for two my size
  8   Out of control temporarily.
  9   Out of control consistently.
 10   Body is plagued with chronic health risks from long-term over-eating.

Then, when selecting and eating food, imagine your control panel and adjust it to how you feel currently, how you choose to feel during the eating process, and how you choose to feel when you're all done eating and drinking. Enjoy the freedom that self-management offers.

Caloric Intake and Use

Everything that you eat or drink becomes "you" for either a short or lengthy duration of time. Thus, you are what you eat. This means that the food nutrients you eat are used to maintain basic body functions such as breathing, blood circulation, normal body temperature, and growth and repair of all tissue and are related to fixed factors such as age, body size, and physiological state. Any kind of caloric intake that your body doesn't use or doesn't eliminate through solid or liquid waste is kept and worn as body fat for future energy needs. Thus, if you don't use it, or eliminate it, you *wear* it!

Caloric Expenditure

Every moment of every day, no matter what activity you are engaged in, from sleeping to aerobically exercising, you are using up calories. Caloric energy expenditure is most influenced by how physically active you are all day. The body's basic needs are more or less fixed, but the amount of physical exertion in which you engage is a personal decision.

How physically active your life is depends on your choice of profession and your choice of recreational activities.

It all depends upon a multitude of day-to-day choices: whether to walk to the local store or drive the car; use the stairs or elevator; rake the leaves or hire it done; go out for a bicycle ride after supper or watch a TV show. How physically active your life is depends as much on attitude as it does on opportunity.[25]

Formula For Weight Maintenance

If you can imagine a picture of the concept of "energy in" and "energy out" balanced, you can then understand maintenance, or staying the same weight. To remain at the same weight, you must intake the amount of calories you expend every day.

How much energy you eat and expend every day to stay at your current weight is determined next.

Figuring Weight Maintenance[26]

A.   Record your present weight, in pounds:
B.   Record your type of life-style; number values are:
    12 — sedentary
    15 — active physically
    18 — pregnant/nursing
    20 — varsity athlete or physical laborer
C.   Multiply A times B:

This is your weight maintenance number, or the number of calories per day you need to eat to stay at your current weight.

Caloric Expenditure for Various Activities

How many calories you burn per minute during any activity depends upon two criteria:

▶ The *intensity* at which you perform the exertion (high-, medium-, or low-level work or exercise).

▶ Your body weight.

The higher the intensity, the more calories you burn per minute. For example, you expend more energy and calories running a mile than you do walking that mile. And the heavier you are, the more calories per minute you will burn. (Just like full-size cars burn more fuel per mile than the small compact models.)

Caloric Intake Needed To Gain Lean Weight

The caloric requirements to add one pound of body muscle is 2,500 calories. (This includes about 600 calories for the muscle, and the extra energy needed for exercise to develop the muscle.) Thus, the daily caloric excess, over your maintenance number just figured, is 360 calories.[27]

You must first, however, be at or below your ideal weight to go on an excess calorie eating program to gain muscle. You want to use your excess body fat first for your energy requirements.

To gain: 1 pound of muscle gain
2,500 calories equivalent of 1 pound of muscle,
÷ 7 days in a week
= 360 daily excess calories to eat, over maintenance intake number

---

Note: Taking in more than 1,000 calories per day over the number needed to maintain weight is likely to result in weight gain as body fat, even if you are exercising strenuously on a regular basis.[28]

Caloric Intake Needed To Lose Body Fat

It is physiologically impossible to lose more than two to three pounds of body fat per week.[29] A weight loss greater than this will represent water and lean body tissue. You'll look lousy, feel weak, be hard to live with, and you will inherit every germ floating by you, when you drop your lean weight.

To systematically drop that unwanted extra body fat, you need to drop 3,500 calories a week, or 500 per day, to lose one pound of body fat per week.

To lose: 1 pound fat
3,500 calories
÷ 7 days per week
= 500 calories a day less than your maintenance number

Note: If you desire to drop more pounds per week, but the total caloric intake would be less than 1,200, you need to re-establish your goal or lose only one pound per week. You never want to eat fewer than 1,200 calories per day. A daily diet of less than 1,200 calories is likely to be deficient in needed nutrients for you to grow, repair, stay well, and have energy to perform daily tasks and leisure. Sometimes on a one-to-one basis, a doctor will prescribe a patient to eat fewer than 1,200 calories per day, but he or she will provide extensive guidelines and supplementation. This is *only* under strict supervision of a doctor.

Again, to lose one pound of fat per week, you need to eliminate 500 calories every day. This reduction can be accomplished by either eating less or exercising more. But remember, for say one hour of aerobics (including the warm-up, aerobic movement, cool-down, and relaxation), you will only use up approximately 300 calories. Is it realistic to think that every day you will engage in more hours of endurance exercise than you now do? It's highly unlikely for the average individual. Therefore, eliminating 500 calories should predominantly be by eating less food. If you have yet to develop a fitness program, of course, your elimination of 500 calories per day would come from both the increased intensity and time duration of your exercise, and eating less.

SUMMARY OF WEIGHT MANAGEMENT

To maintain a specific weight, your caloric input must equal your caloric output to be balanced.

To gain or lose weight, there must be an imbalance of energy. To lose fat, the expenditure has to be a greater number because it takes a loss of 500 cals. per day to lose 1 lb. of fat To facilitate gaining lean, the intake has to be a greater number because it takes adding 360 cals. per day to gain 1 lb. of muscle.

To provide a continual means of self-discipline concerning your weight control:

▶ Assess your weight (Chart 12) whenever any major gain or loss has occurred to your lean or fat weight;

▶ Continue setting short and long range goals to achieve or maintain your ideal weight;

▶ Monitor your weight for changes especially if you are prone to having difficulty keeping your weight maintained at your ideal.

Taking time to educate yourself about how to control your weight can be a very interesting experience.

It will provide you with a basis of understanding how the human body physiologically works and how it doesn't work. You can then be alert to all of the false notions, especially of weight loss, that are rampant today. You can develop a program that will work for a lifetime.

GOAL SETTING STRATEGIES

Your program is complete. You have both physical fitness and mental training strategies on the how to become fit and how to maintain that fitness. It's time to challenge yourself, establish your priorities, and then set your program goals.

Priorities

Priorities are the means to reach your goals. They are how you spend your time. Make a list of your top 10 time priorities — how you actually spend your mental and physical energies each week. Identify a rank order as to what time spent is most-to-least important to you. Record any time-robbers that take you away from the priority. Can you identify a role model of excellence who you associate with this priority?

Goal Setting

Goal setting will require you to ask yourself a few questions so that exciting, achievable goals can be set.

ESTABLISHING PRIORITIES

PRIORITIES are the means to your ends (i.e., goals). They are things you give TIME to in the wellness areas of your physical/social/emotional/philosophical-spiritual/intellectual/talent expression dimensions.

– 1 – TOP 10 PRIORITIES	– 2 – ROLE MODEL	– 3 – HOURS GIVEN EA. DAY	– 4 – HOURS GIVEN EA. WK.	– 5 – TIME ROBBER	– 6 – RANK ORDER OF IMPORTANCE:
					#
					#
					#
					#
					#
					#
					#
					#
					#
					#

1. Step one is to become clear as to what result(s) you'd like to experience. Ask yourself, "What will I see, hear, feel in regards to results?" You'll recognize these are the components of motivation.

2. Ask yourself why you are totally committed to achieving each goal. Involve your values now to answer this question. Values are any of the following: adventure and change, commitment, freedom, pleasure to others, happiness, health, love, power, prestige and worth, security, life purpose, success, talent expression, trust or loyalty.

3. Break the link of the old programmed ways by asking yourself what painful values do you choose to avoid. Some of these pain-avoidance values are: anger or resentment, anxiety or worry, boredom, depression, embarrassment, frustration, guilt, humiliation, jealousy, overwhelm, physical pain, prejudice, rejection, sadness.

4. Now re-establish the pleasure link by picturing, hearing, feeling actions you choose to take or do immediately in each goal area to chunk away at mastering each goal. What is something you can start doing right now and within the next 24 hours?[30]

First, this goal-setting procedure tells your brain directly what exact goal you are choosing to set. Second, solid reasoning is provided for why you're etching this goal-set groove deeper. Third, this procedure will break old programming by presenting your pain-avoidance reasons. And fourth, positive action choices are made immediately to create the motivational pictures, self-talk, and movements necessary to initiate active change in your program. It would be helpful to once again make an audio-tape for yourself, on which the goal questions were fully answered. The guidelines for making and playing it are similar to those identified in Chapter 1.

SUMMARY — GOAL SETTING STRATEGIES

Goals, when they are properly internally set and continually nourished, will become reality. Believe it and you will see it. Your future resides within you as a rich resource of possibilities. Enjoy tapping into that unlimited potential.

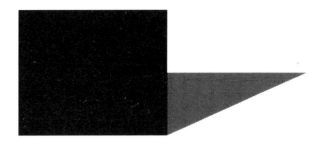

References

Chapter 1

1. Prather, Hugh, *there is a place where you are not alone* (New York: A Dolphin Book, Doubleday and Company, Inc., 1980), p. 96.
2. Helmstetter, Shad, Ph.D., *What To Say When You Talk To Yourself* (New York: Pocket Books, Simon & Schuster, Inc., 1986).
3. Robbins, Anthony, *Unlimited Power* (New York: Fawcett Columbine, 1986), p. 19.
4. Ibid., p. 155.
5. Andreas, Connirae, Ph.D., et.al., *Heart Of The Mind* (Moab,Utah: Real People Press, 1989); Robert Dilts, et.al., *Neuro-Linguistic Programming: The Study of the Structure of Subjective Experience* (Cupertino, CA: Meta Publications, 1980); David Gordeon, et.al., *The Neuro-Linguistic Programming Home Study Guide* (San Rafael, CA: FuturePace, Inc.)
6. Prudden, Suzy, *IDEA Today,* "Affirmations Work!", April, 1991, p. 57.
7. Robbins, Anthony, *Unlimited Power* (New York: Fawcett Columbine, 1986), p. 31.

Chapter 2

1. Paffenbarger, Ralph, et.al. *New England Journal of Medicine*, Vol. 314, No. 10, March 6, 1986.
2. Cooper, Kenneth H., M.D., M.P.H., *Running Without Fear.* (New York: M. Evans and Company, Inc. 1985), p. 195.
3. "Still peddling exercise. Ken Cooper targets kids, older adults." *USA Today*, 7 August 1991, sec. D., p. 2.
4. Cooper. *Running Without Fear*, p. 195.
5. Parsons, Terry W. "Positive Lifestyle Strategies," quoting Dr.Kenneth Cooper's research. Lecture to 'Anchor Fitness Course', September 18, 1990.
6. Kenneth H. Cooper, Movie, "Run Dick, Run Jane." Brigham Young University, Provo, Utah. 1971.
7. Cooper, Kenneth H., *The Aerobics Way.* (New York: M. Evans and Company, Inc., 1977), p. 10.
8. National Vital Statistics Division, National Center for Health Statistics, Rockville, MD, 1988.
9. American College of Sports Medicine 1990: Position Stand, "The Recommended Quality and Quantity of Exercise for Developing and Maintaining Cardiorespiratory and Muscular Fitness in Healthy Adults." *Med. Sci. Sports Exerc.* 22.2, pp. 265-274, 1990.
10. Cooper,Movie, "Run Dick, Run Jane", 1971.
11. Zohman, Lenore R., M.D., et.al., *The Cardiologists' Guide to Fitness and Health through Exercise* (New York: Simon and Schuster, 1979), p. 72.
12. *The Harvard Medical School Health Letter.* Volume X, No. 6, April 1985, p. 3.
13. Ibid.
14. Ibid.
15. ACSM Position Stand, 1990.
16. Ibid.
17. Ibid.
18. Ibid.
19. Ibid.
20. Unpublished research data of Karen S. Mazzeo collected on students enrolled in aerobic dance courses, 1984–1986.
21. Borg, G. A. V., "Psychophysical Bases of Perceived Exertion." *Medicine and Science in Sport and Exercise* 14, 1982.
22. "Rules on Exercise Start To Change." *The Sunday Denver Post/Contemporary*, 30 September 1990, p. 22.
23. Williams, Charlotte A. "THR versus RPE. The debate over monitoring exercise intensity." *IDEA Today*, April 1991, p. 42.
24. Ibid.
25. Ibid.
26. Bowling Green State University Student Recreation Center *Fit-For-All* Manual, 1991-1992, p. 31.
27. Williams, p. 42.
28. Williams, p. 40.
29. Williams, p. 42.
30. Alan, Ken. "A Choreography Primer." *IDEA Today*, January 1989.
31. Francis, Lorna et.al. "Moderate-Impact Aerobics." *IDEA Today*, September 1989.
32. Francis, Lorna et.al. "Injury Prevention. Low-Impact Aerobics: 'Do's and Don'ts'." *Dance Exercise Today*, Nov./Dec. 1986.

33. Ibid.
34. Alan, Ken, "A Choreography Primer." *IDEA Today*, January 1989.
35. Francis, Lorna et.al. "Moderate-Impact Aerobics." *IDEA Today*, September 1989.
36. Francis, Lorna. "Injury Prevention. Combination Aerobics." *Dance Exercise Today*, May 1988.
37. Francis, Lorna. et.al. "Moderate-Impact Aerobics." *IDEA Today*, September 1989. Also in *Aerobics Choreography* (San Diego: IDEA, The Association for Fitness Professionals, 1990).
38. Candace Copeland Videotape, *The Low-Impact Challenge For The Fitness Professional*. (Newark, N.J.: PPI Entertainment Group/Parade Video, 1991).
39. Francis, "Moderate-Impact Arobics," 1989.
40. Copeland videotape, 1991.
41. Francis, "Moderate-Impact Aerobics," 1989.
42. Ibid.
43. Ibid.
44. "Research: Caloric Expenditure in LIA vs HIA" from study, 'The Metabolic cost of Instructor's Low Impact & High Impact Aerobic Dance Sequences.' *IDEA Today*, January 1991, p. 8.
45. "Tempo and Ground Reaction Forces for LIA and HIA" from study 'Comparison of Forces in High & Low Impact Aerobic Dance at Various Tempos'. *IDEA Today*, May 1991, p. 9.

Chapter 3

1. Questions taken in part from the PAR-Q developed by Dr. Richard W. Bowers, Director of the Fitwell Program, BGSU Student Recreation Center, Bowling Green, Ohio; "Taking the Chance Out of Fitness Assessment," *IDEA Today*, June 1991, p. 42; and Personal Excellence™ Consulting Agreement. "Exhibit C: Responsibilities of Client", developed by John M. Dunipace, Atty. and Karen S. Mazzeo.
2. Cooper, Kenneth H., M.D., M.P.H., *Running Without Fear*. (New York: M. Evans and Company, Inc., 1985), p. 128.
3. Ibid, p. 192.
4. Ibid, p. 197.
5. Cooper, Kenneth H., M.D., M.P.H. *The Aerobics Program for Total Well Being*. (New York: M. Evans and Company, Inc., 1982), p. 141.
6. Ibid.
7. Ibid.
8. Zohman, Lenore R., M.D., et. al., *The Cardiologists' Guide to Fitness and Health Through Exercise*. (New York: Simon and Schuster, 1979), p. 87.
9. R.V. Hockey, *Physical Fitness: The Pathway to Healthful Living*. (St. Louis: Times Mirror/Mosby College Publishing, 1985).
10. Hoeger, Werner W. K., *Principles & Labs for Physical Fitness & Wellness*. (Englewood, CO: Morton Publishing Company, 1991), p. 133, 135.
11. Hoeger, Werner W. K., *Lifetime Physical Fitness and Wellness*. A Personalized Program. (Englewood, CO: Morton Publishing Company, 1986), p. 47.
12. Hoeger, *Principals & Labs for Physical Fitness & Wellness*, p. 80.
13. Ibid, p. 83.
14. Ibid, p. 84.
15. Ibid, p. 85.
16. Ibid, p. 90.

Chapter 4

1. Candace Copeland-Brooks Videotape, *Moves . . . and More!* (San Diego, CA: IDEA, Inc. 1990).
2. Candace Copeland videotape, *The Low-Impact Challenge For The Fitness Professional*. (Newark, N.J.: PPI Entertainment Group/Parade Video, 1991).
3. Julie Moo-Bradley & Jerrie Moo-Thurman videotape, *Aerobics Choreography in Action: The High-Low Impact Advantage*. (San Diego, CA: IDEA, Inc. 1990).
4. Lynne Brick videotape, *Total Body Workout*. (Philadelphia: Creative Instructors Aerobics, 1991).
5. Jones, Amy. "Point-Counterpoint. Sequencing a Dance-Exercise Class." *Dance Exercise Today*, May/June 1985.
6. American College of Obstetricians and Gynecologists: *Safety Guidelines for Women Who Exercise* (ACOG Home Exercise Programs). Washington, D.C., ACOG, 1986, p. 6.
7. Hesson, James L. *Weight Training For Life*. (Englewood, CO: Morton Publishing Company, 1985), p. 33.
8. Ibid.
9. SPRI Products, Inc., 507 N. Wolf Road, Wheeling, IL 60090. *Pumping Rubber*, (instructions for product use) 1988. 1-800-222-7774.
10. Ibid.
11. Ibid.
12. Ibid.
13. John Patrick O'Shea, *Scientific Principles and Methods of Strength Fitness*, Second Edition. (Addison-Wesley Publishing Company: Reading, Mass., 1976), p. 89.
14. Kravitz, Len MA. et. al. "Static & PNF Stretches." *IDEA Today*, March 1990.
15. Ibid.
16. Ibid.
17. Ibid.
18. Price, Joan MA. "Stepping Basics." *IDEA Today*, November/December 1990. p. 57.
19. Kravitz, Len MA. "The Safe Way To Step." *IDEA Today*, April 1991, pp. 47-50.
20. Sports Step, Inc. videotape accompanying The Step, *Introduction To Step Training*, (Atlanta: 1989).
21. Lynne Brick, R.N. & David Essel, M.S. videotape, *Pump N' Step*, 1991.
22. Francis, Lorna, Ph.D.; Francis, Peter, Ph.D.; and Miller, Gin. *Step-Reebok. The First Aerobic Training Workout with Muscle. Instructor Training Manual*. Reebok International Ltd., 1990.
23. Ibid, p. 6.
24. Ibid, p. 16.
25. Ibid, p. 17.
26. Ibid.

27. Cooper, Kenneth H., M.D., M.P.H. *The Aerobics Program for Total Well-Being* (New York: M. Evans and Company, Inc., 1982), p. 129.
28. Ibid, p. 144.
29. Level I Walking Only Program written by Dr. Richard W. Bowers, ACSM certified Program Director, Fitwell Program, Student Recreation Center, Bowling Green State University, Bowling Green, Ohio. 1990.
30. Hargarten, Kathleen, M.D., "A Rope-Jumping Class," *IDEA Today*, March 1989.

Chapter 5

1. Zohman, Lenore, M.D., et. al., *The Cardiologists' Guide to Fitness and Health Through Exercise* (New York: Simon and Schuster, 1979), p. 81.
2. Ibid, p. 87.
3. American College of Obstetricians and Gynecologists: *Safety Guidelines for Women Who Exercise* (ACOG Home Exercise Programs). Washington D.C.: ACOG, No. 2, 1986, p. 6.
4. Richie, Douglas H., Jr., D.P.M. "How To Choose Shoes." *IDEA Today*, April 1991, p. 67.
5. Ibid.
6. ACOG, No. 2, p. 5.
7. Ibid., pp. 4-5.
8. Orthotic for sports shoe prescribed and dispensed by Dr. Charles Marlowe, Podiatrist to Karen S. Mazzeo, summer 1983, with accompanying brochure of information.
9. ACOG, No. 2, p. 5.
10. Committee on Nutritional Misinformation, Food and Nutrition Board, National Research Council, National Academy of Sciences, "Water Deprivation and Performance of Athletics." distributed by the Nutritional Education and Training Program, Bowling Green State University, 1981.
11. American Alliance for Health, Physical Education, and Recreation. *Nutrition for Athletes. A Handbook for Coaches.* (Washington, D.C.: AAHPERD, 1971), p. 42.
12. American Alliance for Health, Physical Education, Recreation and Dance. *Nutrition for Sport Success* (Reston, VA: AAHPERD), 1984, p. 2.
13. The American College of Sports Medicine. *Encyclopedia of Sports Sciences and Medicine* (New York: The Macmillan Company, 1971), p. 215.
14. Ibid, p. 216.
15. *The Harvard Medical School Health Letter*, Volume VIII, No. 2, p. 4.
16. The American College of Sports Medicine, p.216.
17. Interview with Jane Steinberg, Athletic Trainer of Intercollegiate Sports at Bowling Green State University, Bowling Green, Ohio, Spring 1982.
18. American College of Obstetricians and Gynecologists: *Safety Guidelines for Women Who Exercise* (ACOG Home Exercise Programs). Washington, D.C., ACOG, 1986, p. 6.
19. Interview, Steinberg, 1982.
20. The Harvard Medical School Health Letter, Volume XI, No. 5, p. 4.
21. Cooper, Kenneth H., M.D., M.P.H. *Running Without Fear.* (New York: M. Evans and Company, Inc.), 1985, p. 128.

Chapter 7

1. Francis, Lorna Ph.D.; Francis, Peter Ph.D.; and Miller, Gin. *Step-Reebok. The First Aerobic Training Workout with Muscle. Instructor Training Manual.* Reebok International Ltd., 1990.
2. IDEA. *Aerobics Choreography.* San Diego: IDEA: The Association for Fitness Professionals, 1989.
3. Ibid.
4. Mazzeo, Karen. *et. al., Aerobic Dance - A Way To Fitness, Second Edition* (Englewood, CO: Morton Publishing Company, 1987) p. 112.
5. Ibid, p.113.
6. Kravitz, Len M.A., and Rich Deivert, Ph.D., A.T.C. "The Safe Way To Step." *IDEA Today*, April 1991, pp. 47-50.
7. Francis, Lorna Ph.D., et. al. pp. 23-25.
8. Ibid, p. 25.
9. Ibid.
10. Sports Step, Inc. videotape accompanying The Step, *Introduction to Step Training* (Atlanta: 1989).
11. American College of Sports Medicine 1990: Position Stand, "The Recommended Quality and Quantity of Exercise for Developing and Maintaining Cardio-respiratory and Muscular Fitness in Healthy Adults." *Med. Sci. Sports Exercise* 22:2, pp. 265-274, 1990.
12. Sports Step, Inc. videotape.
13. Hesson, James L. *Weight Training For Life* (Englewood, CO: Morton Publishing Company, 1985), Appendices pp. 164-165.
14. SPRI Products, Inc., 507 N. Wolf Road, Wheeling, IL 60090. *Pumping Rubber* (instructions for product use), 1988. 1-800-222-7774.
15. Lynn Brick, R.N. & David Eassel, M.S. videotape, "Pump N' Step, 1991.
16. SPRI Products, Inc. & Brick Bodies videotape *Step Strength*. (Wheeling, IL: SPRI Products, Inc.).

Chapter 8

1. Webster's New Twentieth Century Dictionary Unabridged, Second Edition. (New York: Simon and Schuster, 1983) p. 319.
2. Copeland-Brooks, Candice, "Smooth Moves." *IDEA Today*. June 1991, p. 34.
3. Price, Joan. "Open The Door To Men." *IDEA Today.* February, 1989.
4. Platus, Julie "Theme Classes." *IDEA Today.* November/December, 1988.
5. Francis, Lorna, Ph.D.; Francis, Peter, Ph.D.; and Miller, Gin. *Step-Reebok. The First Aerobic Training Workout With Muscle. Instructor Training Manual.* Reebok International Ltd., 1990, p. 6.

Chapter 9

1. Cooper, Kenneth H., M.D., M.P.H. *The Aerobics Programs For Total Well-Being,* (New York: M. Evans and Company, Inc. 1982), p. 141.

2. Power, John S. J. *Why Am I Afraid To Tell You Who I Am?* (Allen, TX: Tabor Publishing, 1969), p. 56.

3. Roman G. Carek, Ph.D., Director of the Counseling and Career Development Center, Bowling Green State University, Bowling Green, Ohio, from his Stress Management presentation in the LIFE Seminar Workshop Series, 1982, held at the Student Recreation Center of BGSU.

4. Taken in part from technique developed by Dr. Bernie Rabin, psychologist and lecturer to Karen S. Mazzeo's Personal Wellness, Health Methods, and Stress Management classes from 1980-1988, Bowling Green State University, Bowling Green, Ohio.

5. Adapted from an original "Natural Highs" model, given to Karen S. Mazzeo's Personal Wellness class, Bowling Green State University, Bowling Green, Ohio, 1988, by an anonymous student.

Chapter 10

1. Nutrition Education Services/Oregon Dairy Council, 10505 SW Barbur Blvd., Portland, Oregon 97219 pamphlet, "Super FOUR, A Star-Studded Guide To Food Choices", 1991.

2. Tillapaugh, Judy, R.D. "Cross-Training in the kitchen." *IDEA Today*, October, 1991, p. 21.

3. National Dairy Council, "Guide to Wise Food Choices" B 170-1 (Rosemont, IL: National Dairy Council, 1978), p. 4.

4. National Dairy Council, "Guide to Good Eating-A Recommended Daily Pattern" B 164-5 (Rosemont, IL: National Dairy Council, 1980), 4th Edition, 1977. A revised pamphlet visual is available, "Guide to Good Eating", 0001N3 1991 (Rosemont, IL: National Dairy Council, 1989), 5th Edition, 1991.

5. In-service seminar for Health Education Division Faculty of School of Health, Physical Education, & Recreation, Bowling Green State University, Bowling Green, Ohio, December, 1990, given by nutrition education consultant Jan Meyer of Dairy and Nutrition Council, Mid East, Toledo, OH.

6. Nutrition Education Services/Oregon Dairy Council, "Super FOUR" pamphlet.

7. National Dairy Council, "Guide to Wise Food Choices," p. 4.

8. Ibid.

9. Nutrition Education Services/Oregon Dairy Council, "Super FOUR" pamphlet.

10. Jan Lewis, "Nutrition Notes: Nutrition and the Athlete" Workshop Series, Nutrition Education and Training Program, Bowling Green State University, Bowling Green, OH, 1981.

11. Nutrition Information and Resource Center, The Pennsylvania State University, Beecher House, University Park, PA, pamphlet "Vegetarianism Throughout the Life Cycle."

12. Jan Meyer, DNC consultant, inservice seminar, December 1990.

13. Tufts University Diet and Nutrition Letter, "Special Report. More than 100 frozen dinners worth heating", Vol. 8, No. 2, April 1990, pp. 3-6.

14. Ibid.

15. Tufts University Diet and Nutrition Letter, "Special Report. Water, water everywhere, but is it fit to drink?", Vol. 9, No. 1, March 1991, pp. 3-6.

16. Ibid.

17. Ibid.

18. U.S. Department of Agriculture, U.S. Department of Health and Human Services, Home and Garden Bulletin No. 232, "Nutrition and Your Health, Dietary Guidelines for Americans", Third Edition, 1990.

19. Lucy M. Williams, M.S., M.Ed., R.D., lecture and literature, "Shopping Tips For Low Fat, Low Salt, Low Cholesterol Diets", delivered to Karen S. Mazzeo's Anchor Fitness-Personal Excellence class, February, 1991.

20. Ibid.

21. U.S. Department of Agriculture, "Nutrition and Your Health, Dietary Guidelines for Americans", 1990.

22. Jan Lewis, "Nutrition Notes. Dietary Guidelines 2," Bowling Green State University, Bowling Green, OH, 1981.

23. Andreas, Connirae, Ph.D., Andreas, Steven A., M.A. *Heart Of The Mind* (Moab, Utah: Real People Press, 1989), p. 251.

24. Ibid, p. 125.

25. Lewis, "Nutrition Notes. Dietary Guidelines 2", p. 6.

26. Cooper, Kenneth H., M.D., M.P.H., *The Aerobics Way.* (New York: M. Evans and Company, Inc., 1977), p. 142.

27. Lewis, "Nutrition Notes. Dietary Guidelines 2", p. 4.

28. Ibid.

29. Ibid.

30. Anthony Robbins audio-tape series, "Personal Power," Robbins Research International, Guthy-Renker Corporation, 5796 Martin Rd., Irwindale, CA 1989.

APPENDIX

Index Card of Information —
A Profile on You

In order to maintain a profile on students who enroll in a class, it is important to keep a few statistics so that change can be noted and statistics developed for future reference. Please fill in the following information, remove carefully from the textbook, and give to your instructor.

NAME _____ RANK:F/So/J/S/Grad/Other

ADDRESS_____PHONE _____

SOCIAL SECURITY NO. _____AGE_____HEIGHT_____WEIGHT_____IDEAL WEIGHT _____

RATE YOUR FITNESS LEVEL: **SUPERIOR/EXCELLENT/GOOD/**FAIR/POOR/VERY POOR-PRE
SUPERIOR/EXCELLENT/GOOD/FAIR/POOR/VERY POOR-POST

PREVIOUS CLASS OR INSTRUCTION IN COURSE: _____

SPORTS IN WHICH YOU PARTICIPATE/ENJOY ON A WEEKLY BASIS: _____

REASON(S) FOR TAKING COURSE:_____

DID ANYONE RECOMMEND THIS COURSE OR INSTRUCTOR? _____

PHYSICAL LIMITATIONS _____

FOLD OUT HERE

ACTIVITY THAT YOU WOULD LIKE FOR ME TO BE SURE TO COVER: _____

HEART RATE: RESTING _____TRAINING ZONE _____

DO YOU TAKE ANY DRUG TO ALTER YOUR HEART RATE?_____

DO YOU DESIRE TO: (CIRCLE) GAIN LEAN WEIGHT / LOSE FAT WEIGHT / STAY SAME

DO YOU SMOKE? _____IF SO, NUMBER PER DAY? _____

RATE YOUR ALCOHOL CONSUMPTION: NEVER / DAILY / OTHER / _____

LIST INTEREST IN MUSIC, FAVORITE SONG, FAVORITE ARTIST: _____

OTHER INTERESTS_____

_____

_____

IF 45 OR OLDER, OR HAVE SPECIFIC LIMITATIONS: I HAVE MY DOCTOR'S WRITTEN PERMISSION TO PARTICIPATE

_____

DOCTOR'S NAME AND PHONE: _____

I have read and understand the responsibilities for participants and the instructor.

_____   _____
              Signature   **Date**

156

CHART 1 SELF MANAGEMENT:
"What Do You Say, When You Talk To Your Self?"

Step I. Have you ever listened to your 'intrapersonal' communication? We talk to ourselves 100% of our waking hours and our internal dialogue is either positive and enabling, or negative and disabling to us.

What do YOU say when you talk to yourself? Become aware and listen to yourself for an hour, a day, or two days, and write your internal dialogue statements (both positive and negative) on this chart.

Our self-talk usually takes the form of "I" statements followed by: "am / enjoy / hate / fear / think / feel / want / need / worry about / " etc.

Examples:

▶ "I enjoy Peter and his attention to details."

▶ "I have been such a klutz! I've dropped everything today."

▶   ▶

▶   ▶

▶   ▶

▶   ▶

▶   ▶

▶   ▶

▶   ▶

▶   ▶

▶   ▶

▶   ▶

▶   ▶

▶   ▶

▶   ▶

Note: Staple any additional sheets to this assessment.

Step II. After you've recorded all of your Self-Talk for several days, go back and evaluate each comment as positive or negative. Circle the ▶ preceding the comment, if it was negative Self-Talk.

Totals: + = _____ − = _____

Step III. After awareness, the next step in re-programming a negative disabling attitude expressed through your self-talk is accomplished by updating and actually re-wording each negative statement you wrote down so that each reads as positive and enabling to you. This opens a main channel for you to begin to achieve your goal of attitude improvement.

1. A listing of negative language you are replacing includes all of the following past or future tense verbs and adverbs (ie., in regards to personal attitude and fitness mindset improvement): need to, want to, ought to, should, could, wish, used to be, and was.

2. Re-write each of the predicate phrases, using positive, *present-tense* language (I am; I enjoy; I can; and use verbs with 'ing' on them as much as possible) and state them as if you have *already achieved* the outcome of the new script you're choosing to program.

   Example: Old: I need to quit smoking.
   New: "I *enjoy being* a non-smoker."

3. You can *add another* helpful line or two, to each new script, if you wish.

   Example: Old: I need to cut out eating high fat, high salt, and highly sugared foods like cookies, for snacks when I get hungry mid-morning at work.
   New: "I enjoy selecting a highly nutritional, low calorie snack like fruit or juice when I get hungry at work mid-morning. *I feel better about myself every time I make this better choice.*"

4. It is best to state positives of positives. However, if you choose to add the negative because you think it will help, place it as the second or *last sentence* of your new script.

   Example: Old: I need to exercise more than once a week, and eat less junk food like donuts.
   New: "I am exercising 3 miles everyday and enjoy being a 'fat-burner' instead of a 'fat-storer'." *I never eat FAT PILLS (donuts) any more!*"

5. Be very *specific* as to the outcome of each new scripts' goal. Tell your brain exactly what you want and are now choosing to do!

   Example: Old: I enjoy exercising to improve my health.
   New: "I enjoy exercising for *40 continuous minutes, 4 or more days every week,* to continue achieving my goal of *dropping a pound of body fat a week.*"

CHART 2 SELF MANAGEMENT:

Observing the "Self-Speak" of Others

Step I. Begin to be aware of *what other people say outloud about themselves* (to themselves, or to another person who's around). Listen for what they think, want, need, see, hear, feel about anything they talk about.

Step II. Also listen for **who** is influencing or controlling the person or, **what** basic **need** has programmed that particular self-speak in the person's life. For example, who = parent, boss, teacher, friend, mate, religious leader; need expressed = power/prestige/talent expression/self esteem; **or** variety and change in life; **or** health/wellness/to physically stay alive; **or** love/emotional or social belonging; **or** spiritual/intellectual growth, etc.

Step III. Record on this assessment the person you observe; what you hear them say; who/what seems to be in control; and assess if the Self-Speak is positive and enabling to the person, or negative and disabling to the person.

Observed Person's Name/Relationship	Self-Speak They Stated:	Who/What Is In Control:	Positive Negative
Examples:			
▶ Susan Smith	"I can't do that move!"	Esteem	Negative
▶ John Jones	"Darn! I need to lose ten pounds yet to play!"	Coach	Negative
▶			
▶			
▶			
▶			
▶			
▶			
▶			
▶			
▶			
▶			

CHART 3 SELF MANAGEMENT:

Listening To & Observing "Media-Talk"

Step I. Listen, observe, and then list examples of "media-talk" from radio, TV, newspapers, magazines, etc., and record how you have in the past, or are now, responding to it.

Source of "Media-Talk":	Programmed "Media-Talk' Message Given:	Your Response: Physically / Socially / Emotionally / Intellectually / Spiritually / Talent Expression Used:
Example:		
IDEA Today 1/91/p.77	"If obesity remains untreated in childhood, only one in 28 children will maintain a normal weight as an adult."	Volunteer my time (talent expression) to a local grade school to endurance exercise (by pace walking) with children, four days a week, for 40-60 continuous minutes.
▶		
▶		
▶		
▶		
▶		
▶		
▶		
▶		
▶		
▶		
▶		
▶		

CHART 4 SELF MANAGEMENT:
"Beliefs / Philosophies By Which You Live."

Step I.   Make a list of your favorite beliefs, quotes, slogans, or philosophies by which you live, that you truly believe and follow. They are everywhere around you — on your classroom and office walls, bumper stickers on your car, slogans on your tee/sweat shirts, and philosophies you quote throughout the day. Staple additional pages to this assessment as your list grows.

Examples:

+ / ⊖   "Too many cooks spoil the broth!"

+ / ⊖   "I never run well on cold days. My muscles cramp up."

⊕ / −   "This moment is a fresh, new opportunity. The past does not equal the future." (Tony Robbins)

⊕ / −   "The only definition for 'failure' is when I stop trying something altogether. I've reprogrammed all other ideas of failure (when I don't get what I wanted or needed) to mean I received 'feedback' / 'results'."

⊕ / −   "Dirty deal situations and experiences happen, and they serve us and help us to grow." (If this is hard to accept, personalize it and ask yourself, what is the worst life experience I've ever had—what long range benefits did it give to me? Didn't I grow a lot afterwards?)

⊕ / −   "It is much more empowering to notice what we can control, and use that to get what we want, than to feel helpless about what we cannot control." Connirae & Steve Andreas

▶

▶

▶

▶

▶

▶

▶

▶

▶

▶

▶

▶

▶

Step II.   After you've recorded your beliefs, go back and evaluate each as either positive ⊕ and enabling to you, or negative ⊖ and disabling to you for developing your full, unlimited potential mindset.

Step III. Re-programming your negative disabling beliefs by which you live: Re-word each belief you wrote down that was negative and disabling, so that each now reads positive and enabling to you. This opens the channels for you to achieve your goals.

Examples: "People are my greatest resource! When a lot of people want to be in charge (too many cooks), I give each one a special important responsibility that contributes to the team effort (broth)."

"Since I can't control the weather, I control my reaction to it. I mentally warm up all my muscles as I stretch, saying, 'My muscles are lo-o-n-g, w-i-d-e, and w-a-r-m. I am ready to run and do my best in this race!"

▶

▶

▶

▶

▶

▶

▶

▶

▶

Step III.

CHART 5 SELF MANAGEMENT:

Making Your Own Re-programming-For-Improvement Tape On Your Behaviors, Emotions, Attitudes & Beliefs

The development of your very own "Tape Talk" tool can prove to be one of the most influential and quickest ways for you to achieve changes you're choosing to make. Here are the details.

1. Purchase a good, blank audio-tape cassette that is at least 30 minutes in length on a side. Give it an interesting title!

2. Review your self-management self-talk assessments and take note of some of the most used negative self-talk ideas or phrases you use (Chart 1, Steps I/II/III). Select 10 re-programmed scripts (Step III) to tape.

3. The remaining 5-8 new programmed scripts you tape can be the re-worded beliefs/philosophies that you listed (Chart 4, Step III). Or, it can include beliefs new to you that you choose to adopt, that haven't "stuck" yet. Remember to use positive, present tense language throughout.

4. Take your written-out, prepared new scripts, and on the tape, repeat each of the suggestions 3 times, with a short pause in between each suggestion.

5. Repeat this procedure for each new script. (If you have 15 new scripts, there will be a total of 45 suggestions; if you use 18 new scripts, there will be 54 new suggestions.)

6. End the tape session by recording each of the phrases/scripts one more additional time each, but this time change "I" to "You". This provides for the external validation that we all need to have. The total number of scripts on your entire tape will now be the total of 60/72.

   Example: "I am a good listener and enjoy hearing what others have to say" becomes . . . "You are a good listener and enjoy hearing what others have to say."

7. If at all possible, add appropriate instrumental music while you tape. Soft, pulsating music seems to affect the way the brain receives and permanently stores information. In order to do this, you'll need an additional tape player, playing the music on it separate from your taping instrument.

8. Talk your scripts onto your tape with emotion! Any programming you currently have in your head is and has been more permanently etched if you experienced it in a highly emotional state.

9. Remember to enjoy re-working your thoughts in language you will enjoy hearing! This is a lot of fun, and just wait until you begin experiencing the results! It is exciting how quickly it can all happen, if you are faithful in playing your tape with regularity.

10. Play your tape while you are doing something else — getting ready each morning, during a break while you are relaxing, during a drive in the car to or from class or work, or as you are getting ready for bed. Play it once or twice a day the first three weeks; then once a day until you realize . . . I've mastered these! It's time to make a new tape on other new challenges!

Planning Page.

▶

▶

▶

▶

▶

▶

▶

▶

▶

CHART 6

Plotting Your Resting Heart Rate

Establishing RsHR

WEEK 1:

Day 1: _____

Day 2: _____

Day 3: _____

Day 4: _____

Day 5: _____

Sum Total: _____

÷ 5: _____ RsHR

Week		II		III		IV		V		VI		VII		VIII		IX		X	
Class	1	2	1	2	1	2	1	2	1	2	1	2	1	2	1	2	1	2
Bi-Weekly Resting Heart Rate																		
120																		
115																		
110																		
105																		
100																		
95																		
90																		
85																		
80																		
75																		
70																		
65																		
60																		
55																		
50																		
45																		
40																		
35																		
30																		

NOTE: Take your resting heart rate at the first possibility in the A.M., before arising. Use first two fingers at thumb side of wrist, carotid artery in neck, temple area, or other pulse point.

Resting H.R.—Week 1: _____ At Finish: _____ (−)Loss/(+)Gain: _____

CHART 7

How to Figure Your Target Heart Rate Training Zone

Since three basic factors enter into figuring your estimated safe exercise zone, those must be established first:

1. Your current age: _____

2. How active is your life style?_____% MHR. If you are:

   (Choose one:)

   ▶ Non-athletic adult: use 50% of your maximum heart rate.

   ▶ Sedentary: use the figure 60-69% of your maximum heart rate (but only for the first two or three weeks).

   ▶ Moderately physically active: use 70-75% of your maximum heart rate.

   ▶ Active & well-trained: use 80-85% of your maximum heart rate.

3. Your average resting heart rate (established on Chart 6): _____

Now place your numbers in the formula that follows:

A. 220 _____ – _____ = _____**Estimated Maximal Heart Rate (MHR)**
   (Index number)   **(Your Age)**

B. _____ – _____ = _____
          MHR   **Resting HR**   **HR Reserve**

C. _____ × . _____ = _____ + **Resting H.R.** = _____*
   Heart Rate Reserve   **Lower end life-style activity range**
                             (i.e. #2 above)

   _____ × . _____ = _____ + **Resting H.R.** = _____*
   Heart Rate Reserve   **Higher end life-style activity range**
                             (i.e. #2 above)

RANGE

RANGE OF   _____   * This range is your estimated safe exercise zone. Keep your heart
YOUR   rate working in this range while you aerobically exercise for approx-
TARGET   _____   * imately 30 minutes of each session.

                                       Re-figure as you "age," as you can reclassify your "lifestyle" of activ-
                                       ity, or as you have a marked decline in your resting heart rate.

For example: Chris is 20 years old, a moderately active person (70-75% range), with a resting heart rate of 62.

A. 220 – 20 = 200 MHR

B. 200 – 62 = 138 Heart Rate Reserve

C. 138 × .70 = 96 + 62 = 158*
   138 × .75 = 104 + 62 = 166*) Target Heart Rate Training Zone

If Chris keeps working (aerobically exercising) at the range of 158 to 166 heartbeats per minute, the heart would be safely working toward the training effect.

CHART 8

Monitoring Target Heart Rates & Ratings of Perceived Exertion

A. Record six-second or ten-second heart rate counts, for the aerobic intervals you monitor in class. Were you over or under your target heart rate training zone?

	AEROBIC INTERVALS	IN YOUR TRAINING ZONE?	OVER?	UNDER?

WEEK

I. _____ / _____ / _____ /　_____ / _____ / _____ /

II. _____ / _____ / _____ /　_____ / _____ / _____ /

III. _____ / _____ / _____ /　_____ / _____ / _____ /

IV. _____ / _____ / _____ /　_____ / _____ / _____ /

V. _____ / _____ / _____ /　_____ / _____ / _____ /

VI. _____ / _____ / _____ /　_____ / _____ / _____ /

VII. _____ / _____ / _____ /　_____ / _____ / _____ /

VIII. _____ / _____ / _____ /　_____ / _____ / _____ /

IX. _____ / _____ / _____ /　_____ / _____ / _____ /

X. _____ / _____ / _____ /　_____ / _____ / _____ /

B.   Monitoring Your Ratings of Perceived Exertion.*

0.5	1	2	3	4	5	6	7	8	9	10
very very light	very light	light (weak)	moderate	some-what hard	heavy/ strong		very hard			very very heavy almost maximum

*What did you 'feel' during the various segments of your workout hour? During: Warm Up? / Aerobic Segments? / Cool Down? / Relaxation? /

WEEK

I.   _____ / _____ / _____ / _____ /

II.   _____ / _____ / _____ / _____ /

III.   _____ / _____ / _____ / _____ /

IV.   _____ / _____ / _____ / _____ /

V.   _____ / _____ / _____ / _____ /

VI.   _____ / _____ / _____ / _____ /

VII.   _____ / _____ / _____ / _____ /

VIII.   _____ / _____ / _____ / _____ /

IX.   _____ / _____ / _____ / _____ /

X.   _____ / _____ / _____ / _____ /

CHART 9

Your Physical Activity Readiness

NAME _____

ADDRESS _____

Phone (Bus.)_____(Home) _____Age _____Height _____Weight _____

(**NOTE:** The purpose for this questionnaire is to serve as part of pre-screening for both fitness testing and exercise participation. If you respond "Yes" to any question, your instructor will want to talk further to you.)

	YES	NO
1. Has your doctor ever said that you have heart trouble?	_____	_____
2. Do you frequently suffer from pain in your chest or heart, especially with exercise?	_____	_____
3. Do you often feel faint or have spells of severe dizziness? More so with exercise?	_____	_____
4. Has your doctor ever told you that you have high blood pressure?	_____	_____
5. Have you ever been told you have a heart murmur?	_____	_____
6. Has a doctor ever told you that you have a bone or joint problem such as arthritis that has been aggravated by exercise, or might be made worse by exercise?	_____	_____
7. Do you have diabetes mellitus?	_____	_____
8. Are you over 45 and unaccustomed to vigorous exercise?	_____	_____
9. Are you taking any medications or other drugs that might alter your response to exercise?	_____	_____
10. Are you pregnant?	_____	_____
11. Are you a smoker?	_____	_____
12. Have you recently had surgery, are obese, or have special limitations?	_____	_____
13. Do you have an at-risk cholesterol reading?	_____	_____
14. Do you have an abnormal resting ECG?	_____	_____
15. Do you have any family history of coronary disease, before or by age 50?	_____	_____
16. Is there a good physical reason not mentioned here why you should not follow an activity program, even if you wanted to?	_____	_____

If you answered "Yes" to any question, please provide a brief explanation: (Use the back of this sheet if necessary.)

I have answered the above questions to the best of my knowledge.

_____   _____
Signature   Date

CHART 10

Pre- & Post-Physical Fitness Testing and Appraisal Results

Name: _____ Age: _____ Sex: _____

PRE-TEST: Cooper's Twelve Minute and 1.5-Mile Test

A. Cooper Twelve-Minute Run/Walk Test

Start Time:_____ Stop Time:_____ Distance Covered: _____

Check Table 3-1 for Fitness Category.

Circle Fitness Category: Very Poor / Poor / Fair / Good / Excellent / Superior

B. Cooper 1.5 Mile Run/Walk Test

Check Off Laps: (ie., 14 for 190 yd. track; 21 for 126 yd. track):

1 - 2 - 3 - 4 - 5 - 6 - 7 - 8 - 9 - 10 - 11 - 12 - 13 - 14 - 15 - 16 - 17 - 18 - 19 - 20 - 21

Time: _____ OR: Just record here if using an open roadway.

Stop Time: _____

− Start Time: _____

Time: _____

Check Table 3-2 for Fitness Category.

Circle Fitness Category: Very Poor / Poor / Fair / Good / Excellent / Superior

GOAL: _____

POST-TEST: Cooper's Twelve-Minute and 1.5-Mile Test

A. Cooper Twelve-Minute Run/Walk Test

Start Time:_____ Stop Time:_____ Distance Covered: _____

Check Table 3-1 for Fitness Category.

Circle Fitness Category: Very Poor / Poor / Fair / Good / Excellent / Superior

B. Cooper 1.5 Mile Run/Walk Test

Check Off Laps: (ie., 14 for 190 yd. track; 21 for 126 yd. track):

1 - 2 - 3 - 4 - 5 - 6 - 7 - 8 - 9 - 10 - 11 - 12 - 13 - 14 - 15 - 16 - 17 - 18 - 19 - 20 - 21

Time: _____ OR: Just record here if using an open roadway.

Stop Time: _____

− Start Time: _____

Time: _____

Check Table 3-2 for Fitness Category.

Circle Fitness Category: Very Poor / Poor / Fair / Good / Excellent / Superior

GOAL: _____

CHART 11

Pre- & Post-Fitness Testing Muscular Endurance and Flexibility

Name: _____ Age: _____ Sex: _____

SECTION A: Muscular Endurance Testing

Pre-Test

	MEN			WOMEN	
Exercise	**Score**	**% Rank**	**Exercise**	**Score**	**% Rank**
I. Sit-Ups	_____	_____	I. Sit-Ups	_____	_____
II. Push-Ups	_____	_____	III. Static Push-Ups	_____	_____
III. Static Push-Ups	_____	_____	V. Mod. Pull-Ups	_____	_____
IV. Pull-Ups	_____	_____	VI. Fixed-Arm Hang	_____	_____
VII. Bench Jumps	_____	_____	VII. Bench Jumps	_____	_____
	*TOTAL:	_____		*TOTAL:	_____

Average Percentile Rank (divide your *total by 5): _____

Muscular Fitness Score, Classification, and Date: _____

GOAL: _____

Post-Test

	MEN			WOMEN	
Exercise	**Score**	**% Rank**	**Exercise**	**Score**	**% Rank**
I. Sit-Ups	_____	_____	I. Sit-Ups	_____	_____
II. Push-Ups	_____	_____	III. Static Push-Ups	_____	_____
III. Static Push-Ups	_____	_____	V. Mod. Pull-Ups	_____	_____
IV. Pull-Ups	_____	_____	VI. Fix.-Arm Hang	_____	_____
VII. Bench Jumps	_____	_____	VII. Bench Jumps	_____	_____
	*TOTAL:	_____		*TOTAL:	_____

Average Percentile Rank (divide your *total by 5): _____

Muscular Fitness Score, Classification, and Date: _____

*Change experienced from Pre-Test to Post-Test: _____

GOAL: _____

SECTION B: Modified Sit-and-Reach Test > Flexibility Testing

Pre-Test: _____" Percentile Rank: _____ Fitness Classification: _____ Date: _____

GOAL: _____

Post-Test: _____" Percentile Rank: _____ Fitness Classification: _____ Date: _____

Change: _____

GOAL: _____

CHART 12

Body Composition Assessment

SECTION A: Determining Your Percent Body Fat. Record your three skinfold readings, add them together, and record total value.

_____

_____

_____

_____ Total of 3 skinfold readings

Using Table 3-5, 3-6, or 3-7, determine your current percent body fat according to your age and gender and record it here:_____

SECTION B: Determining Recommended / Ideal Body Weight.

1. **Fat Weight:** Multiply your total body weight in pounds (BW) by the current percent fat (%F) you're carrying (see Section A), expressing this percentage in decimal form. (BW × %F). This is your fat weight (FW), the actual number of pounds of fat you now carry. (BW × %F = FW).

2. **Lean Weight:** Subtract your fat weight (FW) from your total body weight (BW − FW). This is your lean weight (LW). (BW − FW = LW).

3. **Select** your desired ideal body fat percentage (IFP), based on your goals and the health or high fitness standards given in Table 3-8. Express this percentage in decimal form.   ._____% (IFP)

4. **Recommended / Ideal Weight:** To calculate your ideal weight, use the following formula:

   LW % (1.0 − .IFP) − Recommended / Ideal Weight. (IW.)

Example: A nineteen year-old-female who weights 136 pounds and is 25 percent fat would like to know what her recommended / ideal weight should be, with a "desired" fat percentage of 17%, which is high physical fitness standard.

   Sex: female
   Age: 19
   BW: 136 lbs
   %F: 25% (.25 in decimal form)
   IFP: 17% (.17 in decimal form)

1. FW = BW × %F
   FW = 136 × .25 = 34 lbs.

2. LW = BW − FW
   LW = 136 − 34 = 102 lbs.

3. IFP: 17% (.17 in decimal form)

4. IW = LW ÷ (1.0 − IFP)
   IW = 102 ÷ (1.0 − .17)
   IW = 102 ÷ (.83) = 122.9 lbs

5. To reach her ideal weight, she needs to goal-set to loose 13.1 pounds of fat weight (136 − 122.9 = 13 1).

GOAL: _____

CHART 13

Posture Problems: Detecting and Correcting

PRE-ASSESSMENT / POST-ASSESSMENT

BODY SEGMENTS
LISTED HERE
▼

```
┌─────────────┐          ┌─────────────┐
│   ATTACH    │          │   ATTACH    │
│    OWN      │          │    OWN      │
│   SIDE      │          │   BACK      │
│   VIEW      │          │   VIEW      │
│   PHOTO     │          │   PHOTO     │
│   HERE      │          │   HERE      │
└─────────────┘          └─────────────┘
```

SIDE VIEW

1. Body Line: Perpendicular through weight center _____ Zigzags _____

   Therefore is: Balanced_____ Forward_____ Backward _____

2. Head: Up_____ Back, w/chin up _____ Fwd. w/chin forward _____

3. Shoulders: Directly over hip joint _____ Back _____ Rounded, in and forward _____

4. Chest: Balanced w/rib cage lifted_____ High_____ Sags_____

5. Upper Back: Normal curve _____ Concave & accentuated _____ Convex-"humpback;" kyphosis_____

6. Abdomen: Contracted & flat _____ Protrudes _____ Sags _____

7. Lower Back "Lumbar Curve":   Balanced & easy_____ Hollow "swayback"_____ Flat; inclined to the rear _____

8. Pelvis: Balanced _____ Tilted fwd; lordosis _____ Pushed forward_____

9. Knees: Flexed & balanced _____ Forward; too flexed _____ Locked; hyperextended _____

BACK VIEW

1. Body Line: Symmetrical _____ Asymmetrical _____

2. Head: Erect _____ Tilted _____

3. Shoulders: Relaxed, down and level_____ One shoulder high _____(R/L)

4. Upper Back: Straight spine _____ Curves sideward; scoliosis _____

5. Pelvis: Hips level _____ One hip (R/L) high & protrudes_____

6. Knees: Legs straight _____ Kneecaps turn out or in_____

7. Ankles & Body Wt.: Wt. balanced on outer half _____ Roll inward (R/L), "pronated" _____

8. Feet: Parallel w/toes forward_____ Toe in_____ Toe out _____

GOAL: _____

CHART 14

Strength Training with Bands, Tubing, Light (1-4 lb) Free Weights & Tubing with the Bench

Date	Exercise	S / R / Res*	S / R / Res	S / R / Res	S / R / Res	S / R / Res	S / R / Res	S / R / Res	S / R / Res	S / R / Res	S / R / Res	S / R / Res

*S / R / Res = Sets, Repetitions, and Resistance (e.g., 3 / 8 / MT = 3 sets of 8 repet tions with medium tubing).

CHART 15
Creating Your Own Step Training Pattern Variations and Aerobics Exercise Routines

A. Creating Your Own Step Training Pattern Variations

Directions: Following all of the guidelines given in Chapters 4 and 7, create your own patterns, From The End. Remember that for safety reasons only three sides of the bench can be used in a pattern. Start with a bench approach from the end, and proceed incorporating multiple basic step patterns and multiple bench approaches.

1) Indicate the location of the weight-bearing foot (WBF) to start the pattern, freeing the other foot to then be step #1.

2) Begin the pattern by locating a "1" up on the bench (or down on the floor), followed with the location of the next step, identified as "2".

3) Continue on locating steps 3 - 8, then 9 - 16, encircling any step that has a key directive to be noted (ie., ⑧ is a "tap" non-weight bearing move; ⑫ you'll be in an astride position).

4) Identify any "bypass" step movement with a double circle around the weight-bearing foot and labeling the bypass move, (ie., ⑤ fwd. kick).

5) List arm gestures to accompany each step movement, plus any additional choreographed pointers (sounds, etc.) below, at right. Enjoy being creative!

STEPS:

ARM GESTURES TO STEP #:

1. _____
2. _____
3. _____
4. _____
5. _____
6. _____
7. _____
8. _____
9. _____
10. _____
11. _____
12. _____
13. _____
14. _____
15. _____
16. _____

Directions: This worksheet planner is designed to help you become more aware of the unlimited variety of movement possibilities there can be, using the variables for steps and gestures presented in Chapter 8 on choreography.

IMPACT:	LOW-IMPACT													HIGH-IMPACT														
AEROBIC MOVES:	BOUNCING	2FT/HK/'n TAP	1/2 GALLOPING	HOEDOWN	HEEL-TOE	KICKS	KNEE-LIFTS	LUNGING	MARCHING	PACE WALKING	SIDE STEP-OJT	STEP-TOUCH-ES		GALLOPING	HITCH-KICK	HOPPING	SINGLE/DOUBLE	W KICK	W KNEE-LIFT	JOGGING/RUN	JUMPING 2 F.	STRIDE/CLOSED	HOPSCOTCH	LEAPING	POLKA	PRANCING	ROCKING	SKIPPING SLIDING
GESTURE BASICS: ▪BENDING-TWISTING																												
GESTURE STYLE: ▪ATHLETIC-WESTERN																												
ADDED SOUNDS: ▪CLAPS/SNAPS/AUDIB.																												
LEVERS: ▪ARMS SHORT/LONG ▪LEGS SHORT/LONG																												
PLANES: ▪HORIZ./VERT./DIAG.																												
LEVELS: ▪LOW/MEDIUM/HIGH																												
DIRECTION: ▪UP/DOWN ▪RIGHT/LEFT ▪FORWARD/BACK ▪DIAGONAL																												
PATHWAY: ▪STRAIGHT ▪CURVED ▪ZIG-ZAG																												
RHYTHM/BEAT **ACCENTED: 1-2-3-4**																												
SYMMETRY: ▪SYMMETRICAL ▪ASYMMETRICAL																												
FORCE OF: ▪FOOT IMPACT ▪GESTURES																												

CHART 16
Identifying and Fully Using Your Top 20 Resources

Directions: You are invited to identify and fully describe your perceptions concerning your internal resources by:

1 Slowly reading through all of the questions and statements listed here. Do this alone and in a quiet and peaceful place, where you are free to think about your responses.

2 Review the list, then number 1-20, identifying which questions and statements you plan to answer, and then answer them in that prioritized order.

3 Write or tape-record a detailed response to each of these top twenty most important resources (wants, needs, experiences) you have. Allow these responses to be the beginning of your awareness into how resourceful a person you have been, are, and can be! Keep this written/taped detailed response. You will use it to develop relaxation tapes for yourself.

This has proven to be a superior method used to jump right into and begin the journey inward, to self understanding. It helps you to identify strength areas you have mastered, and short suits (weaknesses) you wish to challenge yourself to surface, take a look at, and change to become all you can be. This is the essence of stress/time/life management.

Ponder first, then select your top 20 resources that jump right out at you as being important from the following:

_____ 1. What is the ideal career position and geographical location?

_____ 2. What are your top five priorities, in order of importance?

_____ 3. Who are your heros?

_____ 4. What major goal would you like to accomplish before you die?

_____ 5. Name special talents, hobbies, and/or skills you have.

_____ 6. What are your positive stress outlets?

_____ 7. What are your negative (poor choice) stress outlets and health habits?

_____ 8. What is the first thing you do when you wake up in the morning? And, what is the last thing you do at night, before you go to bed/sleep?

_____ 9. Who dearly loves you the most?

_____ 10. What makes you laugh?

_____ 11. What makes you angry?

_____ 12. What makes you cry?

_____ 13. What do you desperately fear?

_____ 14. Do you enjoy compassionate contact, like hugs, massages, and handshakes?

_____ 15. What health subject do you know a lot about and seem to discuss with others regularly?

_____ 16. What health subject do you know little about and want more information on?

_____ 17. What is your favorite color?

_____ 18. What is your favorite food(s)? Who makes it (each of them) the best?

_____ 19. Where is the perfect place to vacation?

_____ 20. What do you value most in a friendship?

_____ 21. What is your favorite season of the year?

_____ 22. What is your favorite quotation by which you live?

_____ 23. Where do you turn in times of severe crisis?

_____ 24. Do you follow a particular religious faith?

_____ 25. Which one is absolutely necessary, for you to experience love from someone: 1) they show you with gifts or by taking you places; 2) they tell you the words "I love you"; 3) by their touch, you feel it; the key words are ABSOLUTELY NECESSARY?

_____ 26. What do you enjoy singing about?

_____ 27. What type of music relaxes and mellows you? Motivates you and psyches you up? Blows you away, out of control?

_____ 28. Name your favorite all-time best ever song.

_____ 29. Who was your favorite teacher and what characteristic(s) did you most enjoy in him/her?

_____ 30. Do you like yourself?

_____ 31. What is your favorite book and type of reading material?

_____ 32. How do you celebrate birthdays in your family and what was the most memorable one you've ever experienced?

_____ 33. Which holiday is your very favorite?

_____ 34. What do you just hate?

_____ 35. What sports or physical activities do you regularly enjoy?

_____ 36. The physical fitness triangle includes three kinds of activities for a complete and total physical fitness program. Do you have an active program in each component? Which component is your favorite?

_____ 37. Are you physically fit?

_____ 38. Do you consider yourself fat, thin, or ideal in weight?

_____ 39. What is your favorite animated character; cartoon series/character?

_____ 40. Do you eat breakfast? Lunch? Dinner? Which is your biggest meal?

_____ 41. Do you personally know an alcoholic, a drug user, a behavior eating problems person?

_____ 42. Do you speak up when you have been short-changed in the cafeteria or supermarket?

_____ 43. How many brothers and sisters do you have, and where in the lineup are you? Was this an advantage or disadvantage?

_____ 44. Are you adopted? If so, do you know, or choose to know your biological parents?

_____ 45. Are your parents divorced? If so, what age were you when it happened and with whom did you live?

_____ 46. Have you ever experienced (seen) the birth of a baby? An animal?

_____ 47. At what age and circumstance did you first learn about how babies are conceived, ie., intercourse?

_____ 48. Have you ever been physically abused? Sexually abused?

_____ 49. Do you presently have a sexually transmitted disease?

_____ 50. Have you ever been in a traffic accident? Do you wear seatbelts?

_____ 51. Have you ever experienced a medical emergency that required you to give first aid, mouth-to-mouth resuscitation, or cardiopulmonary resuscitation?

_____ 52. Have you ever been in the hospital?

_____ 53. Do you give blood regularly? Have you agreed to be an organ donor?

_____ 54. At what age did you first experience a death or funeral, and what were your remembrances and reactions?

_____ 55. Have you ever known anyone who committed suicide?

_____ 56. Do you have favorite superstitions you follow?

_____ 57. What are your favorite top 3 movies for all time? Actor/actress?

_____ 58. If you could give yourself a label on how you believe you are perceived by others, what would it be?

_____ 59. Where is the safest place in the world that you associate with peacefulness, joy, emotional warmth, and complete relaxation?

_____ 60. If you could ask anyone (a role model of yours/figure in history/instructor of your class/author of _Aerobics_, etc.) one question from the aforementioned list, what would it be?

ENJOY GETTING TO KNOW YOURSELF BETTER AND ALL THE RESOURCES YOU POSSESS!!

CHART 17
Reflecting Upon Your Stress Outlets

Directions:

I.   Read this column slowly & mentally identify if you use this release.

II. Write what stressor would set you off to use this release.

III. How often? *Always; Frequently; Occasionally; Never.*

I. **Frequently Used Stress Releases:**	II. **Stressors Which Trigger Your Need To React This Way:**	III. **Rate Your Usage:**
Alcohol Usage	_____	_____
Become very quiet	_____	_____
Chew gum	_____	_____
Chew your nails	_____	_____
Chew objects (pencils/toothpicks)	_____	_____
Contact (hugs/massages/sports)	_____	_____
Cry	_____	_____
Drink coffee-tea-cola (caffeine)	_____	_____
Draw artistically (masterpieces/doodle)	_____	_____
Drug usage (prescription/illegal)	_____	_____
Eat without monitoring	_____	_____
Exercise strenuously	_____	_____
Expectorate	_____	_____
Get lost in a good book	_____	_____
Go off somewhere to be alone	_____	_____
Hit people	_____	_____
Kick animals	_____	_____
Laugh hysterically	_____	_____
Play a musical instrument	_____	_____
Play loud/soft stereo music	_____	_____
Profanity	_____	_____
Religious resort to prayer/reading	_____	_____
Sex discriminately/indiscriminately	_____	_____
Sleep	_____	_____
Smoke cigarettes/chew tobacco	_____	_____
Take over-the-counter drugs (aspirin/antacids)	_____	_____
Talk on phone	_____	_____
Tease	_____	_____
Throw objects	_____	_____
Write feelings on paper (letters;diary)	_____	_____
Work with your hands (creatively making things)	_____	_____
Yell and scream	_____	_____
Others: _____	_____	_____

IV. Possible Stressful Situations: Select a response from Column I on the other side & write in the blank.

Someone telling you that you need to lose (or gain) weight _____

Studying 5 hours consecutively _____

First awaken in the morning _____

Antics of children or babies _____

Unreasonable roommate/spouse activity _____

Watching four TV "soaps" in a row _____

See an advertisement for a "binge" food _____

Parental/ or Spouse pressure (grades, money) _____

Fail exam/course _____

Watching an exciting sports event in person _____

After a tedious 8-hour work day _____

Receiving a huge parking fine _____

Long lines _____

Before a speech _____

Waiting for a long overdue (late) friend _____

Budgeting your bills _____

Cleanliness of room/roommate (spouse) _____

Messiness of room/roommate (spouse) _____

Hearing unjust gossip about yourself _____

After a heated argument _____

Negative criticism of your efforts _____

In the company of strangers _____

Must do before you go to sleep _____

Note: Place an asterisk (*) by the negative stress releases you use and wish to improve upon or totally change.

V. What I've learned about myself and my positive and negative reactions to stressful situations:

VI. One resolution or goal:

CHART 18

My Daily Consumption

DATE/ TODAY	/	/	/	/	/	/
MILK 1						
2						
MEAT 1						
2						
FRUIT & VEG. 1						
2						
3						
4						
GRAIN 1						
2						
3						
4						
TOTAL Calories From Above:	1200	1200	1200	1200	1200	1200
Additional Servings Calories:						
Other ("sometimes food") Calories:						
TOTAL DAILY CALORIC INTAKE:						

(a) What groups do you eat with consistent regularity? _____

(b) Which groups do you tend to slight? _____

(c) In which groups and categories do you tend to overeat? _____

(d) Goal: _____

CHART 18

My Daily Consumption

DATE/ TODAY	/	/	/	/	/	/	/
MILK 1							
2							
MEAT 1							
2							
FRUIT & VEG. 1							
2							
3							
4							
GRAIN 1							
2							
3							
4							
TOTAL Calories From Above:	1200	1200	1200	1200	1200	1200	1200
Additional Servings Calories:							
Other ("sometimes food") Calories:							
TOTAL DAILY CALORIC INTAKE:							

(a) What groups do you eat with consistent regularity? _____

(b) Which groups do you tend to slight? _____

(c) In which groups and categories do you tend to overeat? _____

(d) Goal: _____

CHART 19 The Control Panel With One Large Dial

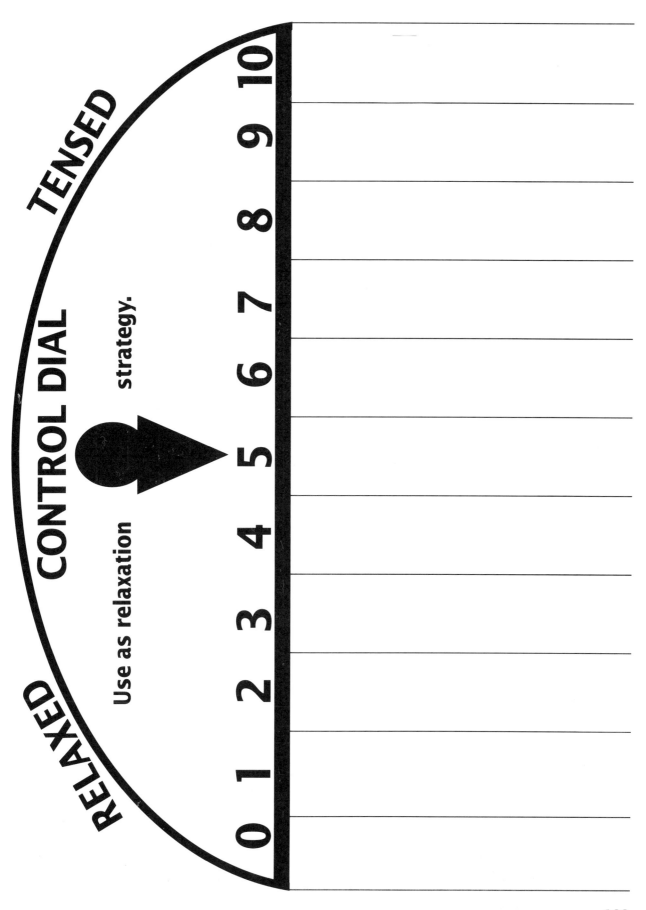

TENSED

RELAXED

CONTROL DIAL

Use as relaxation strategy.

0 1 2 3 4 5 6 7 8 9 10

CHART 20 The Control Panel With One Large Dial

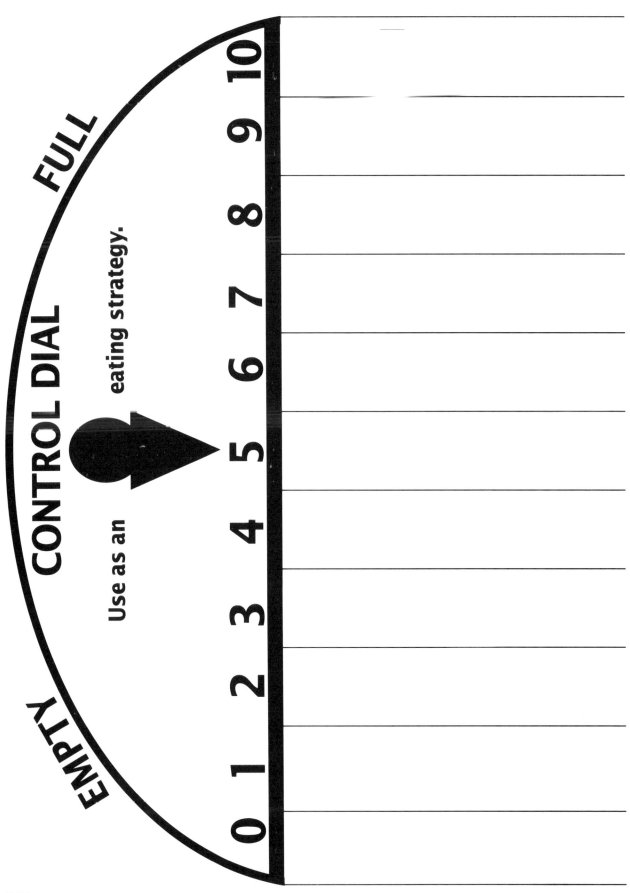

FULL

CONTROL DIAL

Use as an eating strategy.

EMPTY

0 1 2 3 4 5 6 7 8 9 10

Index